THE PRINCESS CHRISTIAN FARM COLONY AND HOSPITAL 1895–1995

"*Just a Bit Barmy*"

THE PRINCESS CHRISTIAN FARM COLONY AND HOSPITAL 1895–1995

"Just a Bit Barmy"

CHRIS ROWLEY

The Author

Chris Rowley was born in Manchester. He read English at Cambridge – sometimes to the surprise of those who have read the proofs of this book. He then went into television, working first in studio management before moving to the scheduling of ITV's programmes. After working in the USA, he moved to programme production, particularly in documentaries, current affairs, drama and news – including producing a BAFTA nominated film on the life of the painter, JWM Turner, "The Sun is God". He moved to the Independent Broadcasting Authority where, amongst other things, he was concerned with the introduction of Channel 4. He was President of The Media Society and a BAFTA judge. He was the Managing Director of a group applying for the Channel 5 licence and was concerned with various local radio stations, including being Chairman of KMFM, the local radio station for Sevenoaks, Tonbridge and Tunbridge Wells. He was the Founder of 'The One World Broadcasting Trust' thirty years ago; Founder of 'The Hand Engravers Association of Great Britain' in 2006/7; and co-Founder of the Heritage Craft Association in 2010. He has written a number of well received books – including a number of short accounts of artists/craftsmen and two books about local history, "We Had Everything ..." and "The Lost Powder Mills of Leigh". For many years he was a long distance runner. He has had a jazz band for over thirty years. He is married to artist/craftsman, Anna Rowley and has two daughters. He lives in the village of Leigh near Tonbridge where he has been Chairman of the Leigh & District Historical Society for many years.

© 2018 Christopher Rowley

A catalogue entry for this title is available from the British Library

ISBN 978-0-9539340-4-1

First edition published in 2018
by Christopher Rowley
Oak Cottage, The Green, Leigh, Tonbridge, Kent TN11 8QL

All rights reserved. No part of this publication may be reproduced in any material form (including photocopying or storing in any medium by electronic means and whether or not transiently or incidentally to some other use of this publication) without the written permission of the publisher.

Design: Amanda Hawkes
Research: Joyce Field
Maps: John Donald
Printed in Great Britain by Lakeside Printing Ltd, Tonbridge, Kent

Dedication

To everyone with whom I have talked – well over a hundred people. All the experts and those who did the caring; and, above all, those very different individuals who needed support, together with their parents. All have been totally helpful, courageous and charming. My thanks.

"One of the highest achievements of a civilization is the way in which it cares for its handicapped members"
PRESIDENT KENNEDY

"I started working at Princess Christian when I was seventeen... Two of the patients particularly touched my heart. One was a smoker and I spent a lot of time teaching him how to catch the bus and pay for the cigarettes... He came back as proud as punch. It was fantastic to have helped him achieve this new level of independence... The other man, a lovely Down's guy, in his late sixties. I used to take him to Rehab and play games and puzzles with him and when he'd [finished his treatment] he'd walk towards me with a huge beaming smile on his face. Three weeks after I left to join the Army, one of the staff phoned me to say he had died. I was heartbroken. But I've never forgotten him. Helping those men towards little improvements in their lives was one of the most rewarding things I've ever done."
KELLY HOLMES

The Princess Christian Farm Colony and Hospital 1895–1995

Some Quotes from the Book

The 1904 architect's drawing shows that the new building was to hold twenty-five feeble-minded boys, a master and a matron.

The term 'mongol', which Dr John Langdon-Down coined in the 1860s was used until the early 1960s when it was renamed Down's syndrome in his memory.

"More nations have sunk to utter insignificance as the result of moral, intellectual and physical degeneracy than by war, famine or any other condition." **1910**

"In the new Boys' Home, they are trained… and in their own dim way, they realize they are of some use and are, therefore, made happy." **1910**

"Every year the newspapers teem with figures demonstrating the increase in feeblemindedness and lunacy… yet the public look on at this rising flood of degeneracy without attempting to stop it…" (**1910 letter to newspaper**).

"GPs in Hampshire used to write NFA on the notes for patients who had what today would be called mild autism. It stood for 'normal for Andover'. **1920/30**

"When we arrived, all the patients would shout 'ello Doctor' and they would hug him and dribble all over him. Then they'd dribble over me too."
Wife of GP, 1960s

"[At Leybourne] I can recall obvious abuse taking place. Pubic hair of women patients was pulled as a way of getting them to comply… But not all aspects were bad." **1970s**

"It is sometimes said – often with distaste – that people who are mentally retarded have a stronger sex drive than the average. Such remarks are annoying because the world is full of people with more or less sex drive than the average."

"I started to prepare for a cooking lesson and some of the staff were horrified. "You can't do that", one said. "You don't know where their hands have been and I said, "Well, I don't know where your hands have been and anyway it's the first thing I'll be teaching them – wash your hands before you start cooking." **1985**

"I remember talking with an elderly lady. She regularly read the newspapers and was very clear-headed. She had been here for years and I asked her how she had come to be at Princess Christian. She told me that her mother had died when she was seventeen and that her father hadn't been able to cope. So she got sent to Princess Christian". **1985**

Some Quotes from the Book

"I had one man who always took his clothes off when he went to the toilet. Once on a trip he said he 'needed to go'. There was no one in the Gents and, as ever, he took all his clothes off. Unfortunately a man came in… He started to say something. I just said, 'Don't worry, it's one of the perks of the job'. He fled." **Nurse, 1980s**

"If you were able to make your own bed, you felt very superior to those who couldn't… One problem was that quite often thunder and lightning made the fire alarms go off. So all the residents were assembled at the fire point. Several times one man was missing – he'd gone back to his room to make his bed." **Nurse, 1980s**

Lady hairdresser: *"It was quite difficult doing a lady's hair with an exuberant man from Princess Christian standing on his head immediately behind me."* **1985**

"You could not impose discipline very easily on those with a learning disability. But if one of them was misbehaving, the punishment could be not being allowed to work with their animals for a time. That worked!" **1990**

"By 1990, with the development of the Villa system, the whole atmosphere could be more relaxed. The staff were not custodians…" **1990**

A couple, both with Down's, were having dinner at an expensive local restaurant. The man got up and knelt in front of the woman and asked "Will you marry me?" "Don't be daft – get up off the floor – and 'yes' of course," she said. **1990**

Fitting into the community is more than people with learning disabilities "learning about life." It also has to be about the community coming half way to meet them. **1990**

"I used to live at Leybourne Hospital – but I'm not naughty now." **1995**

A support worker at a care home: *"I don't think of it as a job. Just me going out each day to meet my friends."* **1995**

"The biggest change in the care of all people in the last thirty years has been the way we look after people with learning disabilities." A GP. **2000**

"Working at the Princess Christian Hospital taught me an awful lot. You don't have to worry and fret about everything in this life." **2000**

Care Home Chief Executive: *"However happy the patients were in an institution, not one would prefer to be back. They like to be out in the real world."* **2010**

Director of KCC Learning Disability Services *"Maybe surprisingly, for me the biggest problem for the future is not funding… it is getting the public to become more understanding."* **2017**

Contents

1 WHAT'S IN A NAME?

From 'Feeble-minded' to 'a Person with Learning Disabilities"	1
Over Three Hundred Names for 'Mad' People	5
Map of where Princess Christian Farm Colony was 1900-1910	10

2 FROM THE START OF AN IDEA TO THE SECOND WORLD WAR

Princess Christian and the Start of An Idea 1896	11
The Conditions the National Association For the Feeble-minded Wanted to Reform	13
The Langdon-Down Family	15
The Foundation of The Farm Colony in Hildenborough 1900-1907	17
Normansfield	21
The First Staff and 'Colonists'	26
Sir Bertram Clough Williams-Ellis	30
The 1911 Census	34
The Formal Opening Planned for 1910 and Further Developments	35
The Girls' Home and the Arrival of Women 'Colonists' 1916/17	37
Work for the 'Boys' in the 1920s	43
Choosing the Farm 'Colonists' in the early1920s	44
Money and the 1920 Fête	47
Death of Jane Langdon-Down 1917 and Reginald's Re-marriage in 1922	51
Oversight of the Colony in the 1920s and 1930s	52
Death of a Resident 1930	53
Medical Treatment 1900-1940	55
Expansion in the 1920s and 1930s	56
1939-1948	59

The Princess Christian Farm Colony and Hospital 1895–1995

The Views of Local Residents 1900-1949   61
The Lack of Records about the Princess Christian Farm Colony   62
Map of Princess Christian Estate 1938   63

3 FROM THE SECOND WORLD WAR UNTIL THE EARLY 1980s

The National Health Service Takes Over   65
Leybourne Grange Hospital 1960-1980   66
The Mental Health Act 1959   71
The Colony Recovers After The War   73
The Princess Christian Hosptital and Its Farm in the 1950s   76
Superintendents and Senior Nursing Officers 1948-1990   83
Life for the 'boys' and 'girls' in the 1960s   89
Farm Managers   91
Problems with the Weather   91
Developments in the 1970s   92
Medical Treatments and Nursing in the 1970s and the early 1980s   94
Administration   106
The Social Club   107
The League of Friends   108
The Position in 1981   112
Maps: Buildings on the Main Site 1980 on   114
       Princess Christian Estate with the Farm 1980 on   115

4 MOVING TOWARDS THE CLOSURE OF PRINCESS CHRISTIAN: 1981-1995

The Inspector Calls: The 1983 Report   117
The Transfer of the Farm from the NHS to Kent County Council   121
The Staff   125
'Care in the Community' Explained   130
How Change was Implemented from Winter 1984/85   131
The Start of the Main Close Down: 1985 on   134
The Introduction of Charitable Sub-Contractors by the KCC   137
Householders' Fears about Mentally Disabled Next Door   139
Funding for the Changes   139
The Final Phases of the Close Down   140
The Carers and Wardens who implemented 'Care in the Community'
      within Princess Christian   144
Spadework   154
The Final Farewell Party   155

Contents

5 CODA: WHAT HAPPENED TO THE BUILDINGS; AND TO THE 'BOYS' AND 'GIRLS'?

The Main Site	157
Glen House	158
Alexander House	159
Hadlow College and the Farm	161
The People's Memories and Views from the Local Community	161
FOOTNOTES	170
HOW THE BOOK CAME TO BE WRITTEN AND ACKNOWLEDGEMENTS	171
APPENDICES	
Appendix 1: A Glossary of Historical Terms for 'Madness'	173
Appendix 2: The National Association for Promoting The Welfare of the Feebleminded	174
Appendix 3: Census Returns for 1911	175
Appendix 4: The future of Leybourne Grange and Princess Christian's by W Cowell, Director of Nursing Services for the Tunbridge Wells Area Health Authority from autumn 1984 issue of Spotlight	180
Appendix 5: Princess Christian Staff Names – primarily post-1945	183
Appendix 6: Princess Christian Material in the Kent Archive	189
NOTES	190
INDEX	198

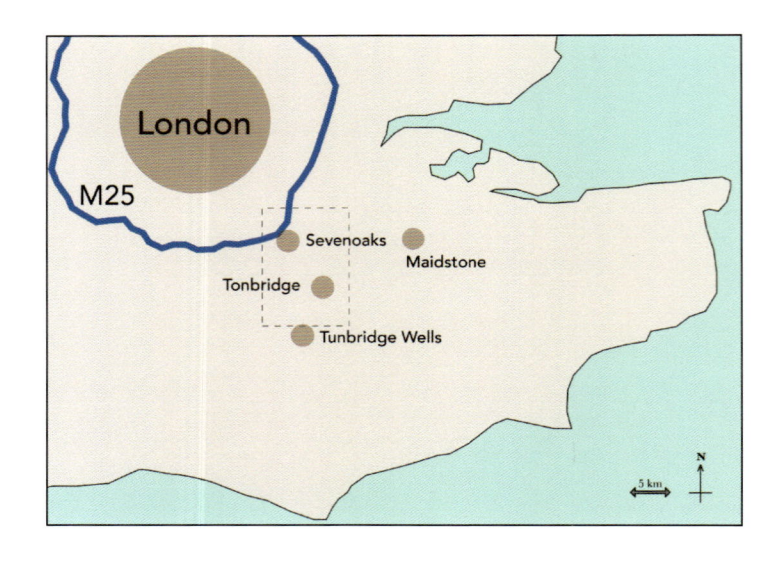

Maps drawn by John Donald

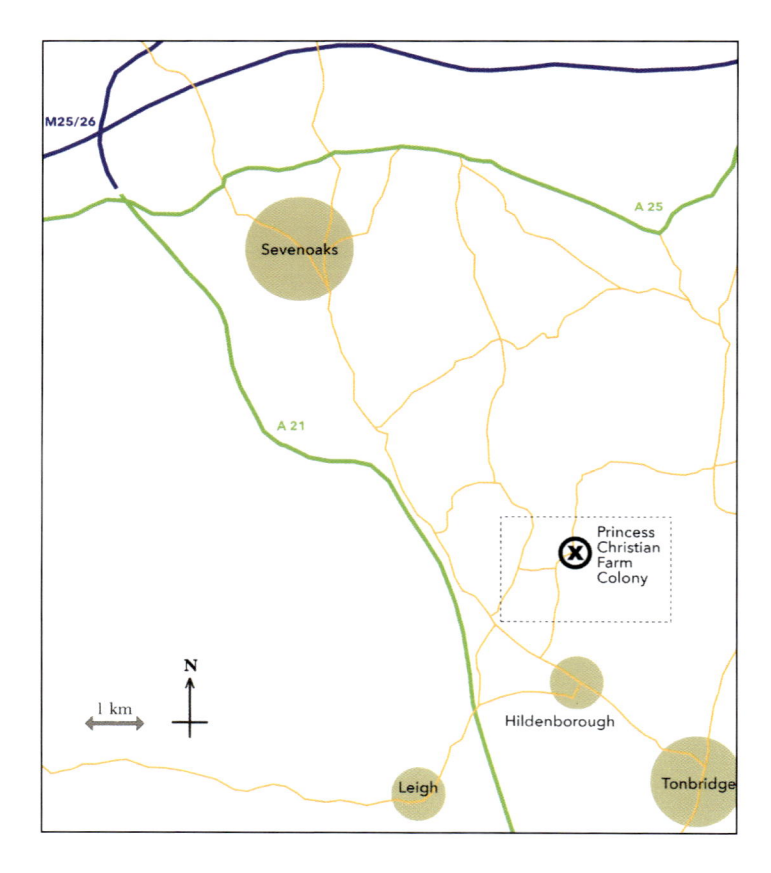

CHAPTER 1
What's in a Name?

From 'Feeble-minded' to a 'Person with a Learning Disability'

Lunatic asylums at the end of Queen Victoria's reign were grim. This book is about an experiment which aimed to look after those who were thought to be lunatics but not too severely lunatic; and to help them in more humane and practical ways. It was not called an asylum. It was called a Farm Colony. And because Princess Christian – third daughter of Queen Victoria – supported the project, it was called The Princess Christian Farm Colony. It was established just outside the village of Hildenborough, near Tonbridge in Kent. These people who were not very mad were known locally as 'barmy', coming from the name of the main lunatic asylum at Barming, not many miles from Hildenborough. So those who were a bit barmy were chosen to live and work at The Farm Colony. However, the medical term for such people was not barmy. It was 'feeble-minded'. This book, therefore, is about what for its first fifty years was known as 'The Princess Christian Farm Colony for the Feeble-minded'.

The Farm Colony ran as a charity from the early 1900s until 1949. At that point, the National Health Service took it over and it became the Princess Christian Hospital before being wound down in 1990-1995. The book shows what daily life was like for those who were almost always called the 'boys' and the 'girls' – whatever their age. It explains how the hundred 'boys' and and fifty 'girls' were looked after not only by the long-serving staff but by the local community. And it explains the difficulties around 1990 of winding down the Hospital, where in many cases the men and women had lived for ten, twenty, even forty years. Then 'Care in the Community' was introduced and the Hospital was closed, with its long-term residents scattered.

The book contains deeply moving material – the stories of the men and women who lived at the Princess Christian Farm Colony and the dedicated staff who cared for them. One of the differences between Princess Christian – as it was usually called – and other lunatic asylums or mental hospitals was partly its size. Because it was so much smaller than the normal asylums, it meant that a family atmosphere was developed and fostered. But it was also unusual in that the problems of those living at the Farm Colony were relatively similar, so they could become part of the community together.

I have heard from around a hundred people – all in their own ways experts – and I am very conscious that I am only a rapporteur, trying to tell the stories of those with whom I have talked. I realise that almost any one of the people I have met could write a whole book about their own experiences. However, what has struck me was not only how different each of the life stories has been but how society's attitude changed over the hundred years 1900 to 2000. The Mental Deficiency Act of 1913 divided people with mental problems into four – 'Idiots', 'Imbeciles', 'Feebleminded' and 'Morally Defective'. A formal description of these and other terms appears in Appendix I, but to the modern reader all these terms seem not only derogatory but overlapping and muddled. For example, 'morally defectives' included people with 'strong, vicious and criminal propensities' – which might seem fair enough. However, it also included 'unmarried mothers' where the family or the village or society were not prepared to help. 'Feeble-minded' was described in the Act as "persons in whose cases there exists mental defectiveness which, though not amounting to imbecility, is yet so pronounced that they require care, supervision and control for their own protection or the protection of others ...."

I had wondered initially whether the book should be called – quoting from the original founding documents of the Farm Colony – 'To help the Feeble-minded' or 'From the Feeble-minded to the Present Day'. The problem with such titles is that, when I consulted other people, they were actively uneasy with even the mention of 'feeble-minded'. They felt that, if the book was intending to show how such people were treated, it might throw a slur upon the people that society was – and is still – trying to help. Increasingly, as the book progressed, it became clear that a term that one generation used to describe people who were somewhat different to the then current view of normality, often changed. What was seen as descriptive and completely acceptable to one generation became distasteful to the next. Professor Steven Pinker invented the term 'euphemistic treadmill' to describe how words or terms changed over time.[1]

What's in a Name?

Before the Victorian urge to erect lunatic asylums in the 1830-1860 period, every village would have had a number of men and women who were called 'slow' or 'soft in the head' or 'simple'. They were seldom dangerous and everyone in the community knew them and accepted them. And, even if the village children probably called them names occasionally, they were a part of everyday life – just a bit different. It was this type of person – as well as a wide range of others – who often were later put into the Victorian asylums.

The Victorians wished to do good. Until then, a village was able (and usually willing) to look after its own 'simpletons' but this was often not practical in the increasingly large towns and cities. The new lunatic asylums, which were built in the early Victorian period, were intended to improve society – to give a proper home to people who were not being cared for in the modern world of the 1830s or 1840s, as well as to house the relatively few unmanageable or dangerous. However, before too long these new asylums became full – often dramatically over full – with a wide variety of men and women, including those who did not fit easily into a respectable Victorian family. Quite a number did not need the confinement which in some cases was imposed upon them. By the end of the century, conditions in the asylums became appalling. There were some doctors who felt it was worth finding ways to help such people; and some who also tried to classify the different types of inmate. Dr John Langdon-Down, an outstanding man in his era, was one of those who aimed to do both. This book has a great deal about his work, and the work of his two sons and their respective wives, who sought to help the 'feeble-minded'. The classification of a certain type of mad or feeble-minded person by Dr John Langdon-Down as 'mongol' lasted as a formal medical term for almost a hundred years before it was re-classified as 'Down's syndrome'[2] in memory of the family. However, from the outset the Langdon-Downs were clear that it was a wider range of men and women for which they would be caring – not just 'mongols'. And care for them they did at the Princess Christian Farm Colony.

In due course, the term 'feeble-minded' was thought to be embarrassing and the authorities invented new definitions. By the 1930s and 1940s there was 'mentally retarded' or sometimes 'mentally defective'. The people living near the Princess Christian Farm Colony had normally got round the problem. They realized they were likely to get the collective name for the Princess Christian residents wrong if they were not careful. So they said the 'boys' and the 'girls' – or occasionally the 'colonists' or 'the people at PC'. By the 1950s and 1960s the authorities were by now using terms such as 'those with mental handicaps'[3] or 'those with mental illness'.[4] The public (including the author) would sometimes say, hoping they had not offended anyone, "he (or she) probably has a mental problem." However, such terminology was soon said to be wrong by the professionals. A mental health problem or mental illness really meant that it was some sort of problem *which could be cured*. These included such things as anxiety or depression, although these then became classified as clinical anxiety or clinical depression. For those who had been born 'different' and *could not be cured* – although they might be helped – the description 'learning disability' became the term which had to be used. However, even there it was possible to get it wrong. I was told: "Some people might say 'a learning disabled person' but we should say 'a person with learning disability'. The person always comes first; then the disability." For some experts, even the word 'disabled' became a term which should not be used; and to say 'he is a Down's syndrome sufferer' or 'an autism sufferer' was also said to be misleading because again "it implied the person had a disease". The terms 'Educational Sub-Normal' and 'Special Educational Needs' and its acronym, SEN, were introduced, particularly in the educational world but have since become frowned upon and 'Additional Needs' has been introduced: 'Autistic Spectrum Disorder' was replaced by 'Autistic Spectrum Condition': and then 'on the autistic spectrum'. Nowadays even to say 'those with Learning Difficulties' has become less welcome, with rather vague phrases such as 'those needing additional help' have become de rigueur. The euphemistic treadmill continues. Today, there are four official types of classification of learning disabilities – mild learning disability; moderate learning disability; severe learning disability; and profound learning disability. These four categories in turn create their own linguistic complexities. There are inevitably many borderline cases which fall between the categories; and, as each category will often entitle the person concerned to different types of assistance, there are disagreements with authorities. Nor do any of these subdivisions even touch upon the illnesses relating to physical disabilities or mental illness.

However, two further problems arise. The first is medical and the second social. On the medical side, every patient is – absolutely rightly – considered an individual, with their own symptoms and behavioural attitudes. Therefore, those caring for them have to have terms which narrow down the specific problem. As medical science has advanced, a whole sub-set of medical diagnostic terms are now used on notes, for example, Williams Syndrome, Rett Syndrome, Prader-Willi Syndrome or one of many dozens of three-lettered acronyms, such as DCD, PDA or PSCN. (Down's syndrome is, apparently, still acceptable to most, but not all, experts).

The second problem is the same old problem: what is the collective noun to use? It is frowned upon to call them 'patients' or sometimes even 'the learning disabled'. In the modern era, the Kent County Council and charitable organizations, which run units or flats where those with learning disability live, used to call the people they looked after 'residents' or 'tenants' – and still often do – but this was thought unfortunate by the authorities; and, in any case, many of the people still live at home or go to Day Centres and use other facilities organized for them. Kent County Council's Social Services Department got round the problem by calling those whom it helps 'service users'.

At this point the author became discouraged. To write a book covering the whole 20th century using 21st century terminology seemed wrong. To refer to these individuals as 'service users' seemed bizarre – although I could see why nowadays the Kent County Council felt the term is not pejorative because it describes the men and women who do indeed use the services provided for them. So, in this first book, I have mainly gone back to the friendly, if often inaccurate, terms used by the staff and the local residents in the 20th century – the 'boys' and the 'girls'. However, whatever 20th century or 21st century collective nouns are used, it should not disguise the major fact that every single person who lived at Princess Christian was a separate individual – and, it seems, with very few exceptions, they were treated as such by the long-serving and dedicated staff.

Three Hundred Different Names for 'Mad' People

As I wrote this book, I started to jot down the names from 'feeble-minded' to 'service user' that have been used for 'mad' people over the last one hundred and fifty years. The problem of giving a name or a classification to types of people who are a bit different is illustrated by the huge number of English words and phrases that have been used. The list that follows of over three hundred and thirty words or phrases can pose two challenges to readers of this book:

- Can you think of even more words?
- Grade them from one to a hundred in terms of what you perceive as the severity of the person's problem. So, perhaps 'psychopath' and 'subhuman' in the top five; and 'barmy' as somewhere near eighty and 'inept' about ninety.

Some of these terms have origins in Greco/Roman words; some originate from Early English, Germanic, Mediaeval and 15th-19th century words and there are a number from rhyming slang (r.s. in the list). There are one or two from India, for example, 'doolally', and a few extras from Ireland and the USA; and typically irrelevant ones from Australia. Increasingly, as society gets more sensitive about labelling people, the formal descriptions get vaguer while the medical terms get more detailed. Perhaps my 'favourites' – for a variety of reasons – are 'differently able' (sounds sensible); 'a kangaroo in the top paddock' (wonderful); NFA and PDDNOS (look at the list for the definitions). Some of the medical terms are given in the list, including a Victorian term, 'West's disorder' – partly because it was named after a local Tonbridge doctor.[5] However, there are many more modern medical terms which have not been mentioned. The wide variety may give some indication that it has always been difficult or embarrassing to categorize those who are different from the ordinary – different from 'us'. So, if you do at least glance down the list, it will remind you of the men and women who, in each generation, needed help and, even more perhaps, needed understanding. It will also lead you into the background of the story of the Princess Christian Farm Colony and the people who tried very hard to make those who lived there feel part of the world around them.

What's in a Name?

Abnormal
Additional needs
Alternative Language Difficulty
Articulation
Aspergers
Attention Deficit Disorder (ADD)
Attention Deficit and Hyperactivity Disorder (ADHD)
Augmentative Communication
Autistic
Autistic Spectrum Condition

Autistic Spectrum Disorder (ASD)
Away with the fairies

Backward
Barking/Barking mad
Barmy
Barmpot
Basket case
Batso
Batty/Bats
Bats in the belfry
Baying at the moon
Bazoodi
Below par
Berk
Berserk

Bi-polar
Blockhead
Bollock Brain
Bonehead
Bonkers
Boob/booby
Borderline Personality Disorder (BPD)
Boron
The 'boys'
Bubblehead
Buffoon
Buggy
Bungalow (i.e. nothing on top)
Buttercup and Daisy (r.s.)

What's in a Name?

Cabbage Head
Case
Central Auditory Processing Disorder (CAPD)
Certified People with Challenging Behaviour
Chump
In cloud cuckoo land
Clown
Clumsy Child Disorder
Cocktail Party Syndrome
Communication and Interaction (C&I)
Compulsive Depressive Disorder
Conduct Disorder
Coot
Crackers
Crackpot
Crack-minded
Crank/cracked
Crazed
Crazy
Cretinous/cretin
Cuckoo

Daffy
Daft
Daft as a brush
Deedle
Defective
Deluded
Dense
Deranged
Developmental Communication Disorder (DCD)
Development Language Disorder
Differently Able
Dickhead
Dilbert
Dilly
Dim
Dimmo
Dimwit
Dink
Dippy
Disabled
Disturbed
Div/Divvy
Doink
Doolally (Indian)
Dope
Dottard
Dotty
Down's syndrome
Dozy
Dromgo (Aust)
Dumb
Dumb-cluck
Dummy
Dunderhead
Dunce
Dungers
Dyscalculia
Dystonia
Dyspraxia

Echolalic
Education, Health and Care Plan (EHCP)
Educationally subnormal
Emotional Disorder
Emotional Stability Personality Disorder (ESPD)
Eros and Cupid (r.s.)
ESN

Feeb
Feeble-minded
A few annas short of a rupee
A few sheep short in the top paddock (Aust)
A few snags short of a barbie (Aust)
A few threads short of a jumper
Flaky (USA)
Fool/Foolish
Fragile X syndrome
Freak
Frenzied
Fruit and nutcase
Fruit cake
Fruity
A fruit-loop
In the funny farm
Funny in the head

Ga-ga
Galoot
Gawnie (Irish)
'My Gentlemen'
The 'girls'
Gone bananas
Goofy
Goon
Gormless

Handicapped
Has problems
Have a screw loose
Haywire
Head basket
High Functioning Disability
Hysterical

Idiot
Idiot-savant
Imbecile
Impaired
An Inadequate
Inept

The Princess Christian Farm Colony and Hospital 1895–1995

Inmates
Insane
Intellectually challenged
Irrational

Jackass
Jughead
"Just call me John?"

A Kangeroo loose in the top paddock
Kanner's syndrome
Keith Moon (r.s.)
Kilkenny Cats (r.s.)
Kit Kat (r.s.)
Klictz
Kookie/kooky

Lakes of Killarney (r.s.)
Lamebrain
Those with learning difficulties
Those with learning disabilities
Those with language impairment
Those with speech and language disorders
Lennox Gastaud syndrome
Lights on but nobody in
Loco
Loghead
Lombard
Loon/Loony
(In the) loony bin
Loopy
Lost his marbles
Low mental order
Lump of school (r.s.)
Lunatic
Lunk
Lunkhead

Mad
Mad as a box of frogs (York)
Mad as a Hatter
Mad as a march hare
Man on the moon (r.s.)
Maniac
Mazawattee
Those with a mental health condition
Those with Mental Health Difficulties
Mental
Mentally defective
Mentally deficient
Mentally disabled
Mentally impaired
Mentally irregular
Mentally retarded
Mentally subnormal
Microcephalic
Microphily
A Misfit
Missing a few cough drops (Suffolk)
Moderate Learning disability (MLD)
Mongol
Monomaniac
Mood disorder
Moonstruck
Morally defective
Moron/moronic
Motor moron
Multiple Personality Disorder (MPD)

NFA (Normal for Andover)
NFC (Normal for Chatham)
Natural Fool
Neuro-atypical

Neurotic
Nincompoop
Nitwit
No one at home
Non compos mentis
Non-verbal
Not all there
Not right in the head
Not quite the full quid (Aust)
Not the sharpest tool in the box
Numskull
Nutcase
'A nut job' (D. Trump)
Nut nut
Nut rock
Nuts
Nutter/nutty
Nutty as a fruit cake

Object prominence
Obsessive Compulsive Disorder (OCD)
Odd
Off his bonce
Off his chump
Off his head
Off his noodle
Off his plonk
Off his rocker
Off his trolley
Of unsound mind
On the autistic s pectrum
On the spectrum
One flew over the cuckoo's nest
One sandwich short of a picnic
One screw loose
One tack short of a tool box (USA)

What's in a Name?

Out of his mind
Out to lunch

Paranoid
Pathological Demand
    Avoidance (PDA)
'Patients'
Pelmans
A penny short of a bob
Persuasive Development
    Disorder (PDD)
Persuasive Development
    Disorder Not
    Otherwise Specified
    (PDDNOS)
Pillock
Plum crazy
Poop
A potato cake short of
    a packet
Potty
Prader-Willi syndrome
Prannock
Pratt
Profound Learning
    Difficulty (PLD)
Profound and multiple
    learning Difficulty
    (PMLD)
Profound and multiple
    learning Disability
    (PMLD)
Profound, severe and
    complex needs (PSCN)
Psychopath

Rabid
Raving
Receptive language
    difficulties
'Residents'
Retardates
Retarded

Rett syndrome
Round the bend
Round the twist

A sandwich short of a
    packed lunch
Scapegrace
Schizoid/schizo
Schizophrenic
Screw loose
Screwy
Self-locked-up Disease
'Service User'
Severe Learning Disability
    (SLD)
Sick in the head
Silly
Simple
Simple minded
Simpleton
Slightly short of East
    Ham (i.e. one tube
    stop from Barking)
Slow
Social Communications
    Disorder (SCD)
Sociopath
Soft
Soft in the head
Spastic
Spackers/spac
Spaz/Spazzer
Special Educational
    Needs (SEN)
Special language
    impairment
Special needs
Speech and language
    disorder
Statemented (of special
    needs)
Subhuman
Stupid

Sturge Weber syndrome
Subnormal
Suitable case for
    treatment
Supportee

Taken to Macclesfield
    (asylum)
'Tenants'
Thick
Thick as two short
    planks
Touched
Troubled
Twat
Two ounces short of
    a pound
Tuppence short of
    a shilling
Turner syndrome

Unbalanced
Unhinged
Unsound
Unstable
Up the pole

Verbal dyspraxia
Village Idiot

Wacky/Whaky
Wacko
Wally
Wazzock
West's disorder
On the Wessex Scale
    (I-IV)
Williams-syndrome

XYY syndrome

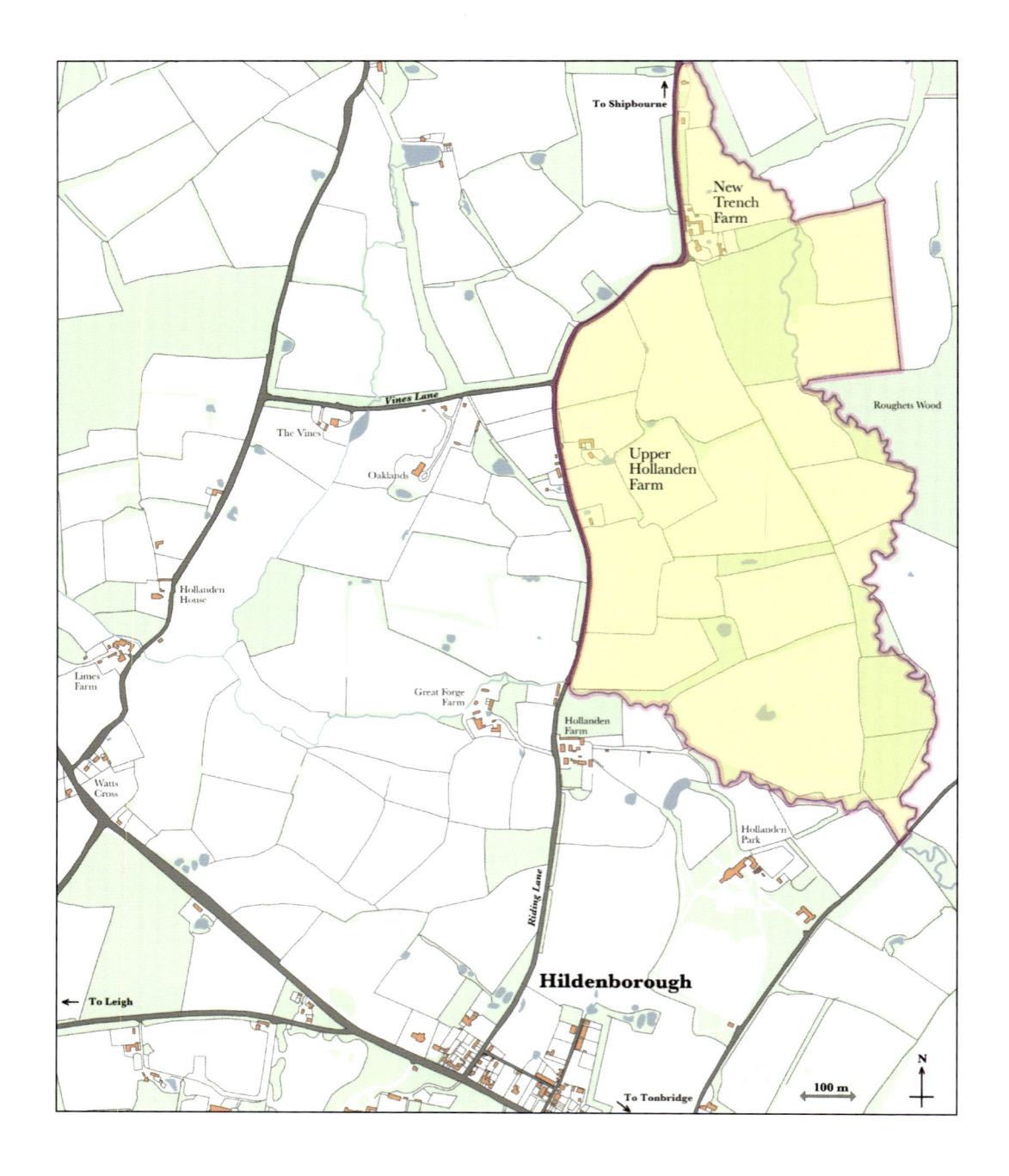

Location of land north of Hildenborough, bought 1900–1908 by Princess Christian Farm Colony from Lord Derby's Estate (in yellow).

Map based on the Ordnance Survey 2nd Edition 1897-1900. Adapted by John Donald.

CHAPTER 2

From the Start of an Idea to the Second World War

Princess Christian and the Start of an Idea 1896

Princess Helena Victoria was the third daughter and fifth child of Queen Victoria. She was born in 1846 and died in 1923. She was always known as 'Lenchen', the Germanic short-form for Helena, in the family. She was described by one historian as 'the most timid of Queen Victoria's children'[6], but that seems surprising. After considerable family opposition, she got her own way and married the penniless Prince Christian of Schleswig-Holstein in 1866. He not only had no money but was also said to look forty-five rather than his actual twenty-five years. As was the custom, she took his family name, becoming Princess Christian. Her marriage should have meant that her home became what is now Denmark but in fact she decided that she and her husband would live in England, near Windsor. This gave her access to her family, particularly the Queen, who we now know was almost impossible in the last thirty-five years of her life. However, her Windsor home enabled her to follow up her various interests in Britain more easily. In fact, she seems to have been the most socially active of Queen Victoria's children. She was one of the founders of the British Red Cross during the Franco-Prussian War and set up various training schemes for nurses which included a nurses' home and training centre in Windsor. She was the President of the Royal Free Hospital Nurses League and was active in helping the St Thomas Hospital Group and its two thousand five hundred nurses. She also seems to have been concerned with improvement in childbirth care. Even when she was elderly in 1919, she founded The Cross Roads Club, which helped mothers and babies; and she was actively concerned with the start of the new British Lying-In

Hospital. Various letters between herself and Florence Nightingale show that they were fighting for the same causes.[7] A ward in the Hospital For Women in London's Soho Square still bears her name; and a training school for nurses and nannies in Manchester named after her was still flourishing until at least the 1960s. There was a Princess Christian Hospital and Sanatorium in Weymouth from 1902 until 1921 when it was absorbed into a larger hospital grouping. Other letters show she was also concerned with the poor – and a new school of art needlework!

Additionally, the Princess brought up her own two daughters to understand their responsibilities in a changing world and they were "grounded in the realities of British medical and welfare work."[8] Her older daughter, Princess Marie Louise, received practical training in First Aid in the field and recalled many years later that, as a six year old, she had been taught to roll bandages for wounded soldiers fighting in the Russo-Turkish War of 1877-1878.[9] So, to a non-expert, Princess Christian sounds an interesting and determined woman.

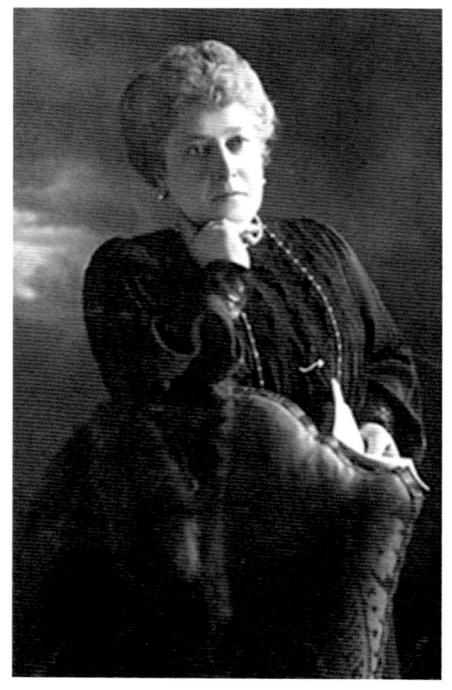

Princess Christian towards the end of her life.
From Wikipedia.

Her connection with the Tonbridge area came later in her life. She had become concerned about mental deficiency and in 1896[10] she became the founding President of a Trust called the 'National Association for Promoting the Welfare of the Feeble Minded'. The Trust's principal aims were to "investigate and spread information about the best methods of ameliorating the conditions of the feeble-minded and to provide homes in the cases in which they seemed necessary". The National Association was also active on the political front and was successful in raising the profile of the less than ideal conditions of the feeble-minded (see Appendix 2 for the official definitions for people who were thought 'mad'). The Association went to lobby Prime Minister Asquith in July 1910[11] and contributed to a change of political and public opinion which in turn led to the Mental

Deficiency Act in 1913. The Association seems to have done good work with school boards too, looking into the best ways to teach children who were feeble-minded. However, this book concentrates on the successful Farm Colony which was established in Hildenborough, near Tonbridge in Kent – the Princess Christian Farm Colony. It was one of the objectives of the National Association to provide accommodation for the feeble-minded. By 1900, the Association had itself set up four small homes for young people of different sexes and ages; and other homes were affiliated to the Association[12]. By 1905 the number of their own homes had risen to twenty-three, with a further fourteen homes affiliated to the Association. However, it seems that the Colony at Hildenborough was the only residential home with a farm that the Association established itself.

The full name of the National Association seems on occasions to have been shortened to the National Association for the Feebleminded and, in later years, both names seemed to be used interchangeably. The situation was made more complex when, before the First World War, a range of like-minded groups joined together to form a new body, the Central Association for Mental Welfare. However, this book will call the original grouping 'The National Association' to cover the variants over the period 1895 to 1948/9. Princess Christian continued to give her support until her death in 1923. Indeed one newspaper reported in 1910,[13] "She had always followed the growth of the Farm Colony with the keenest interest."

The Conditions the National Association Wanted to Reform

The conditions of lunatic asylums towards the end of Queen Victoria's reign were grim. Most had been built in the 1830-1850 period with the best of intentions and at very considerable cost. As we have seen, prior to that period, parishes and families had normally looked after their own, except in very extreme cases. However, with the increasing move of the population to towns and cities, it was difficult to continue the old system of local help. Allied to this urbanization, was the reforming zeal of the period. "Victorian men of influence were united in their vision. The 1845 Lunacy Act directed the mandatory construction of lunatic asylums in every county; and established a Lunacy Commission to regulate them."[14] "A well-run asylum can offer restorative benefits, unavailable to even the most well-meaning family," said one expert in the 1850s.[15] So all counties were required to build asylums, although West Kent's asylum had already been built in 1833 at Barming on the fringes of Maidstone.

It was called the Oakwood Lunatic Asylum and was on a grandiose scale. It had all the mod cons of the age – for example, a steam engine provided heating and ventilation as well as raising the water. It was designed to house one hundred and sixty-eight patients. However, a report eleven years later in 1844 said it now held four hundred and forty-three patients, even if the report also said that Oakwood was one of the better lunatic asylums in the country.[16] Quite clearly in the eleven years since it opened, there had not been a three or fourfold increase in lunatics in West Kent. What had happened – and continued to happen all over the country – was that families or occasionally communities now had somewhere where they could dump a relative or a local who did not fit in; and it was often free too. Conditions almost inevitably became bad.

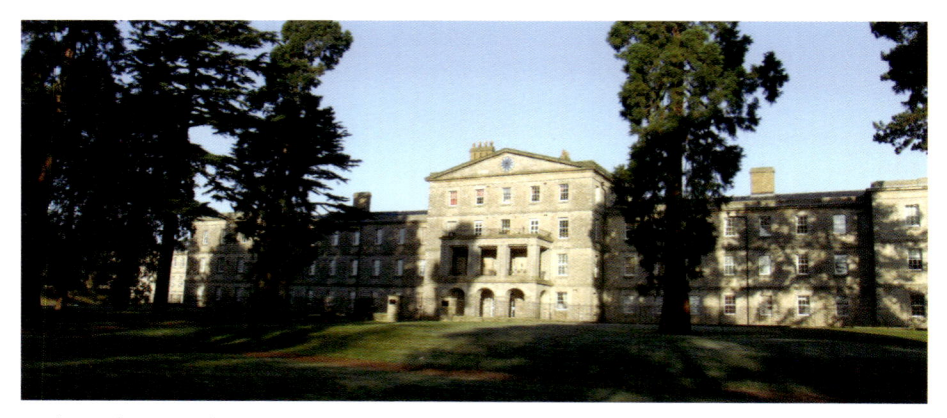

Oakwood Hospital at Barming, near Maidstone, built 1833.
© Moriarty01 / Wikimedia Commons

By the 1870s and 1880s conditions had become much worse. The asylums became full of people whom today we would class as severely autistic and with people who had what today we call Down's syndrome, but also with men and women with moderate or mild learning difficulties, people with slight or severe deformities, epileptics and even with unwanted children and embarrassing unmarried mothers. The state of lunatic asylums by the 1870s and 1880s is described particularly vividly in Sebastian Faulks' novel 'Human Traces'.[17] The building "stretched from horizon to horizon with six miles of corridors." Faulks goes on to tell about the more than two thousand men, women and children, all segregated in wards of up to sixty inmates: the more difficult and even those who complained were in restraints of various types. Funding was inadequate; and staff were in short supply. There could be two or three doctors to look after two thousand inmates and the so-called 'nursing staff' had virtually no training. Some staff tried to be caring but most were ground down, callous and even sadistic. Perhaps worst of all, inmates would not leave until they died – even if they had nothing wrong with them in the first place. It was this type of system that Princess Christian herself and the National Association were trying to improve, certainly inspired by the work of an amazing family – the Langdon-Down family.

The Langdon-Down Family

Dr John Langdon-Down was one of the great Victorian reformers in the field of mental disabilities. Although Princess Christian gave her name to the proposed new Farm Colony, the driving force undoubtedly came from the Langdon-Down family[18], headed by the remarkable father, Dr John. He had been born on 18 November 1828 and baptized at Bethel Chapel at Torpoint, Devon. He was the son of Joseph Almond Down and Hannah Haydon. Joseph had been a grocer – in 1830 Pigots Directory he is given as a grocer, draper and druggist at St Germans, Cornwall. However, he must have done well because he was able to put his son, John, through a medical apprenticeship and then to pay for John's studies when he was a doctor at the London Hospital in Whitechapel – a very poor area of the East End but a much respected hospital. John won a Gold Medal in physiology whilst studying for his MB and took his MRCP and MD degrees. Clearly going far, he was appointed first as an Assistant Physician at the London Hospital but, soon after, as the Consultant Physician to the large Earlswood Asylum for Idiots at Redhill, Surrey. It was here that he seems to have developed his lifelong commitment to those with mental disabilities. He was still a young man, but he decided he would transform the Asylum. The patients at Earlswood would have included people with what today we call autism and 'learning disabilities', but also a good number of people whom society or individual families found embarrassing or difficult to accept. We know from Dr Langdon-Down's own records that he had one patient who could multiply complex figures instantly in his head but could not remember Dr Langdon-Down's name, even though they talked almost every day. There was another patient who had memorized the many volumes of Gibbons 'Rise and Fall of the Roman Empire'. He knew it by heart but did not understand any of it. Dr Langdon-Down accurately analyzed these people and, in doing so, provided what one current expert says "included descriptions that anticipated modern accounts of autistic children… by a century."[19] However, as well as being committed to practical improvements at Earlswood, he was also researching into the different categories of mental illness and in 1866 he published what became a major analysis, 'Observations on the Ethnic Classification of Idiots'. In this he invented the term 'mongol'. His thesis accurately describes the physical characteristics of such people, even if his reasoning of the cause for it was, by later standards, proven wrong. He propounded the idea that, because the physical appearance of such men and women looked like what he thought were people from Mongolia, somehow they had developed what we would today call the genes of Mongolians. He has been criticized for propounding a sort of eugenics but in reality his thesis and his own views were in advance of his time. He did not wish to demean 'his' mongols – indeed he did everything he could to encourage others to help such people; and he was strongly opposed to slavery, denying the theory that the black man was a lower class of human. His general views were liberal and advanced for a Victorian gentleman and he defended the rights of women to higher education, dismissing the then current idea that such education could lead them to be more liable to produce 'feeble-minded' offspring.

However, his major contribution to Victorian society and medicine was the practical care of what he called 'the mentally subnormal' or the 'feeble-minded'. He, and later his two sons, had a vision of something different to an asylum. In 1868 he decided that he would establish his own care home for such people at Normansfield, a large house between Hampton Wick and Teddington on the Thames to the west of London. In 1860 he had married Mary Crellin in Hackney and, until her death in 1901, she was very active as the Administrator at Normansfield. They had two sons, Reginald, born in 1866 at Redhill, and Percival, born in 1868 at Normansfield. Both sons spent their lives, first helping their father run and expand Normansfield until their parents' deaths, after which the sons continued the work at Normansfield and developing the Farm Colony in Hildenborough, with practical ideas to help those who were – in the words of the original Princess Christian proposal – 'feeble-minded'.

Because Dr John was well known in this field, it seems likely that he had met Princess Christian with her own concern for the feeble-minded. When the idea for the Farm Colony was being first discussed, presumably in the mid-1890s, Dr John would have been in his mid-sixties, with his doctor sons both in their early thirties. Together with Dr John's wife, Mary, they would have made an extremely knowledgeable group. However, as the father, John, died suddenly aged only sixty-seven in 1896 and Mary five years later in

From the Start of an Idea to The Second World War

1901, the implementation of the plans for the Princess Christian Farm Colony would have fallen on the younger generation – the two sons, in particular, Reginald. Whatever the early beginning, it does seem likely that Princess Christian was persuaded into the project by the older Langdon-Down generation and was more than happy to encourage Reginald and to a much lesser extent Percival to take the project forward.

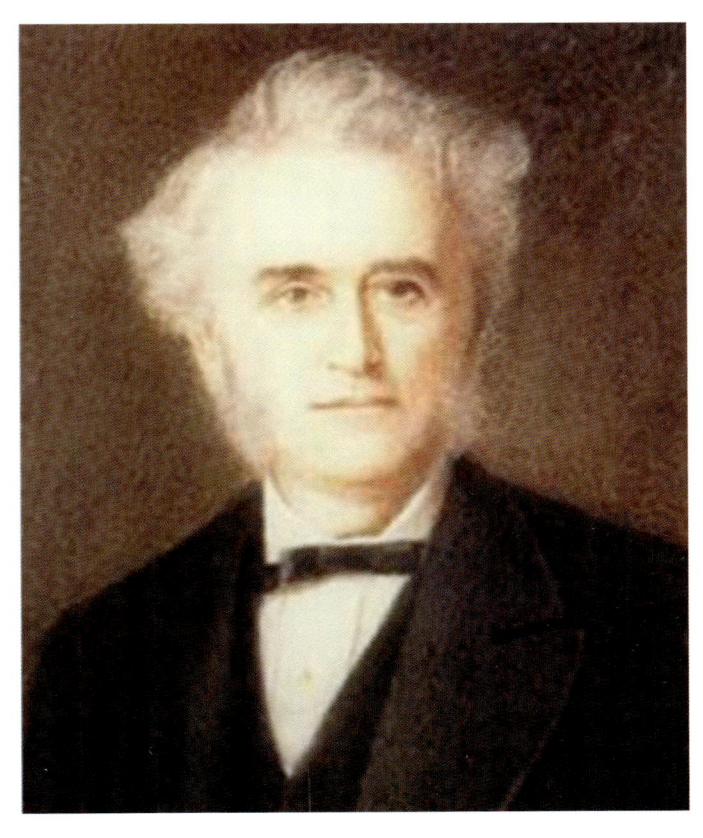

John Langdon Down approx. 1870.
© *Langdon Down Museum of Learning Disability*

The Foundation of the Farm Colony in Hildenborough 1900-1907

It appears that the National Association had been searching without success for some time for a suitable site for a Farm Colony in which to house and help some feeble-minded men and women. It is not clear why Princess Christian and the Langdon-Downs eventually chose to site their Farm Colony in Hildenborough, near Tonbridge in Kent. Neither had any obvious connections with the area as far as we know. One possibility may have been that one or other might have known one of the Lord Derbys whose family was the owner of various pieces of land in Hildenborough.[20] There were three Lord Derbys around this period, Edward the 15th Earl who died in 1893; his brother, Frederick, the 16th Earl who died in 1908; and Frederick's son, Edward Stanley, who then became the 17th Earl. All three were top cabinet level politicians and diplomats and all three moved in the highest levels of Victorian and Edwardian society. Any of the three or perhaps more than one could easily have known Princess Christian and/or the Langdon-Downs in the period when the Farm Colony was being planned. Around the turn of the century, the Derby family owned 70,000 acres of land, much in the North West around Liverpool but also a considerable acreage in Surrey and Kent. The land in South West Kent included over four thousand acres around Hildenborough and to the west of the Shipbourne Road running north from Tonbridge, which included the land on which the Princess Christian Farm was to be established. The majority of the land around Tonbridge and Hildenborough was sold in 1907 but it is not clear whether the sale included the Colony's land – probably not. It seems likely that the land needed for the Colony must have been sold or at least promised to the National Association around the turn of the century because the planning of the buildings started around 1900/1903. Perhaps the various Lord Derbys took a favourable view because of family connections. Edward's grandmother was a Sackville-West at nearby Knole in Sevenoaks; and his mother was very keen on training nurses – a likely link to Princess Christian herself. However, whatever goodwill may possibly have been involved, the Derby estate was not generous about the price. The sale price was £5,000. The land was certainly not a gift, as has sometimes been claimed. The farm initially bought was called New Trench Farm and it was about a mile and a half north from Hildenborough Village on a small road called Riding Lane. At some stage, either with the initial purchase of New Trench Farm or somewhat later, a second adjoining farm, Upper Hollenden Farm was bought. This second property, slightly nearer Hildenborough, became the headquarters for the Princess Christian actual farm, although it was additionally used for some of the accommodation.

Some brief notes on the history of the Princess Christian Colony[21] mention that in 1908 Princess Christian formed a committee for the Hildenborough project. As well as the Royal Princess, the committee was said to have four other members, Dr Reginald Langdon-Down and his wife,

Ruth, his sister-in-law Miss Evelyn Turnbull and Dr Russell Brain. However, the date of this committee must be wrong. In 1908 Russell Brain was twelve years old and certainly not yet a doctor; Dr Reginald did not marry Ruth Turnbull, his second wife, until 1922 when Evelyn Turnbull would have become his sister-in-law. It seems likely therefore that, whilst some sort of committee may have been established in 1908, or even earlier, under the chairmanship of Reginald Langdon-Down with the support of Princess Christian, the three people mentioned above became advisers in the late 1920s and/or the 1930s. Details of these undoubted worthies are given later when covering the 1920/1930 period.

Even if the above committee did not exist until a good time later, there clearly needed to be planning well before the Colony opened. Reginald must have been the driving force behind the plans, particularly after the death of his father in 1896. As we have seen, he had been born in 1866 while his father had been in charge of the Earlswood Asylum and over the next thirty years he had been brought up by a father and mother who had spent their whole lives thinking about and actively caring for the mentally subnormal or feeble-minded. He and his brother, Percival, were both sent to Harrow (In the Harrow School Year Book, Reginald's address is given as 81 Harley Street, his father's consulting rooms, rather than Normansfield. Perhaps he or his family thought that it sounded more respectable to give their father's address in Mayfair rather than an 'Insane Asylum' in Teddington.) In 1886 Reginald went to Trinity College, Cambridge to read Natural Sciences. He obtained a First in Part I. After finishing his three years at Cambridge[22], he then went to the London Hospital where his father had trained and still practised. By 1888 Reginald had done well and ended up with an MB.B.Chir. and by 1894 an MRCP. Maybe just as importantly for this book, at the London Hospital he met a senior nurse, called Jane Jarvie Cleveland. Jane had been born in India in 1864, the granddaughter of a general in the Indian Army and the daughter of the heroic Lt. Colonel, George Cleveland.[23] The family had come back to England sometime in the 1870s and Jane had trained to be a nurse. We do not know any more about her other than she had reached the relatively senior rank of Sister by 1891.[24] Reginald and Jane were married in June 1895 at the fashionable Marylebone Parish Church of St Thomas in Portman Square which was only a few hundred yards from Dr John's consulting-rooms at 81 Harley Street and near to where Reginald eventually had his own private practice at 47 Welbeck Street. Jane's family may have originally been a military one but they became a medical one. Not only was there Jane herself, but her brother, John, went on to become a surgeon and Jane's daughter, Stella, went on to help run Normansfield. Jane's expertise and experience at the London Hospital must have been invaluable to both Normansfield where she became in overall charge of nursing and later as an adviser at Princess Christian. At Normansfield she would have been supervising up to eighteen nurses (female) and twenty-three attendants (male) – as well as at least twenty-four domestic servants who lived on site.[25] So her knowledge would have been particularly useful in the planning and then the working of Princess Christian Farm Colony over the twenty years of her marriage.

To help in the preparatory work at the turn of the century, there was also Reginald's mother, Mary, who had done so much to establish Normansfield and run it on a day-to-day basis. She died in 1901 but she must have contributed a great deal in the initial discussions about the proposed Farm Colony. Reginald would also have been able to call upon the ideas of his younger brother, Percival, who like Reginald had been to Harrow and Trinity College, Cambridge and had trained at the London Hospital before going to work at Normansfield in the mid-1890s. Additionally, as well as all the expertise from family members, there were the other senior staff at Normansfield who would certainly have had an input when the plans for a new Farm Colony were starting, whether it was to do with financial affairs, nursing matters or ideas about what buildings and what ancillary staff would be needed. There was also the National Association, although we have relatively few details about what exactly it did between 1896 and 1920, or how many and what kind of people were initially concerned in the organization. From 1920 newspaper reports, the National Association had Annual General Meetings which were sometimes held at Princess Christian. The Chairman of the National Association for many years was Sir William Chance, Bart (1853-1935), the son of a Midland industrialist and philanthropist who had – as so often in this story – been to Trinity College, Cambridge – albeit some years before the Langdon-Down brothers. He was a well-connected lawyer who became High Sheriff of Surrey in 1911 – a post later held by various gentry from Surrey and even the actress, Penelope Keith, so well known for her upper class roles. We know little more about him or the National Association's various committees until 1921/22 when we have a little more information from the AGM of that year. It is clear, however, that a wide variety of high profile people were concerned with the Association, in part to assist in lobbying; in part to help raise money; and in part to give medical advice.

Although most accounts of the start of the Farm Colony say it was founded or started in 1908 or 1909, the evidence indicates that general planning for it had started well before and some detailed planning had occurred at the turn of the century. The architects' designs for the main boys' house were drawn up in 1904. Those plans for the Hildenborough site could not have been drawn up without at the very least there being an understanding that the land would be available. Nor could the proposal for the land and buildings have been started without some idea of how it would all be financed. While we know little about how the original 1895 Trust was initiated,[26] it seems likely that the Landgon-Down family had detailed discussions both before and after 1895 with the knowledge and general support of the Princess, which would have led to firmer plans and eventually meant that the first buildings were erected or adapted in 1905/6 and the first feeble-minded residents able to arrive at the Princess Christian Farm Colony around twelve months later, probably in 1907/08.

Normansfield

Because we have relatively little about the day-to-day working of the Princess Christian Farm Colony in the first half of the 20th century (the records were apparently thrown out by the NHS in 1949/50), it is worth looking briefly at what was happening at Normansfield.

As we have seen, Normansfield had been started in 1866 by Dr John Langdon-Down and by his wife Mary. One version of history says that it was initially for the 'respectable poor' who could pay little or nothing. Certainly the Langdon-Downs brought some of their patients from the insane asylum at Earlswood. However, another version says it was founded "as a private home for the mentally handicapped, especially for the children of the upper classes." Whatever the case – and it was probably a combination of the two – Normansfield aimed to educate and train the adults and particularly the children in their care to the full extent of their capabilities. The hospital quickly became oversubscribed and the organization expanded, buying more land and from 1872 to 1888 erecting more buildings. In 1879 there were seventy-six male and thirty-five female patients; and in the 1886-1912 period this had increased to an average of a hundred and five men and around forty-five women – roughly the kind of figures for Princess Christian once it became fully established. Expansion at Normansfield not only included more buildings in which the 'patients' or 'residents' lived, but a new drill hall – there were drills on the main parade ground every morning – a theatre and a laundry, together with a boat house on the Thames at the bottom of the estate.

There is a classification of the Normansfield patients' illnesses, with 35% having 'a mental disorder of idiocy and with 65% being described as having 'imbecility'. Appendix 1 explains more fully the range of Victorian terms relating to different types of what today we call 'learning disabilities' but 'idiots' were said to be incapable of guarding themselves against common dangers such as traffic or fire. 'Imbeciles' had less severe problems but their condition still meant that they were unable to manage their own affairs, or, in the case of children, would be unable to learn. And the 'feeble-minded', who had less severe problems still but still needed 'control and supervision' all their lives.

Although we know something about how many living-in staff there were in the early days of Princess Christian from the 1911 census, little is known about the overall staff levels or wages for the first seventy years.[27] However, we do know about Normansfield wages and staffing between 1868 and 1913 from a U3A study (referred to in the notes and available on the Normansfield website.)[28] To give some examples: wages for a twenty-one year old laundry maid were normally around £12 a year, although a housemaid received £17 a year. A nurse aged forty-three who looked after the female patients was paid £20 a year, as was an under-gardener. However, the top of the salary scale – presumably the most difficult person to replace – was the supervisory cook who received £40 a year. (We hardly have a mention of a cook at Princess Christian over of its the whole ninety years.) The hours worked by the nurses and attendants are also given in the U3A study. Shifts averaged twelve hours a day, Monday to Saturday, with a four to eight hour shift one Sunday a month. We can be fairly sure that the wages and the hours at Princess Christian would have been similar.

The staff numbers at Normansfield in both the 1901 census and the 1911 census seem very large. In 1901 there were around ninety-one employees for one hundred and six patients. Even the 1911 census figures show one hundred and twenty-nine patients looked after by seventy-two staff. As well as Reginald himself, who is described as 'resident medical superintendent of the house licensed for imbeciles', there were numerous nurses and attendants, domestic servants and various levels of kitchen staff, medical officers and matrons and a governess of the institution. Even the ratio of 1911 staff to patients seems high when compared to the 1911 census figures for Princess Christian and may indicate that not only were at least some of the patients at Normansfield more difficult but a proportion at Normansfield were paying customers and may have expected more personalized care? The other, more likely, explanation is that the Princess Christian staff figures could well be much higher in reality but, because many or at least some staff lived locally in their own homes, they were not included in the census for the Farm Colony.

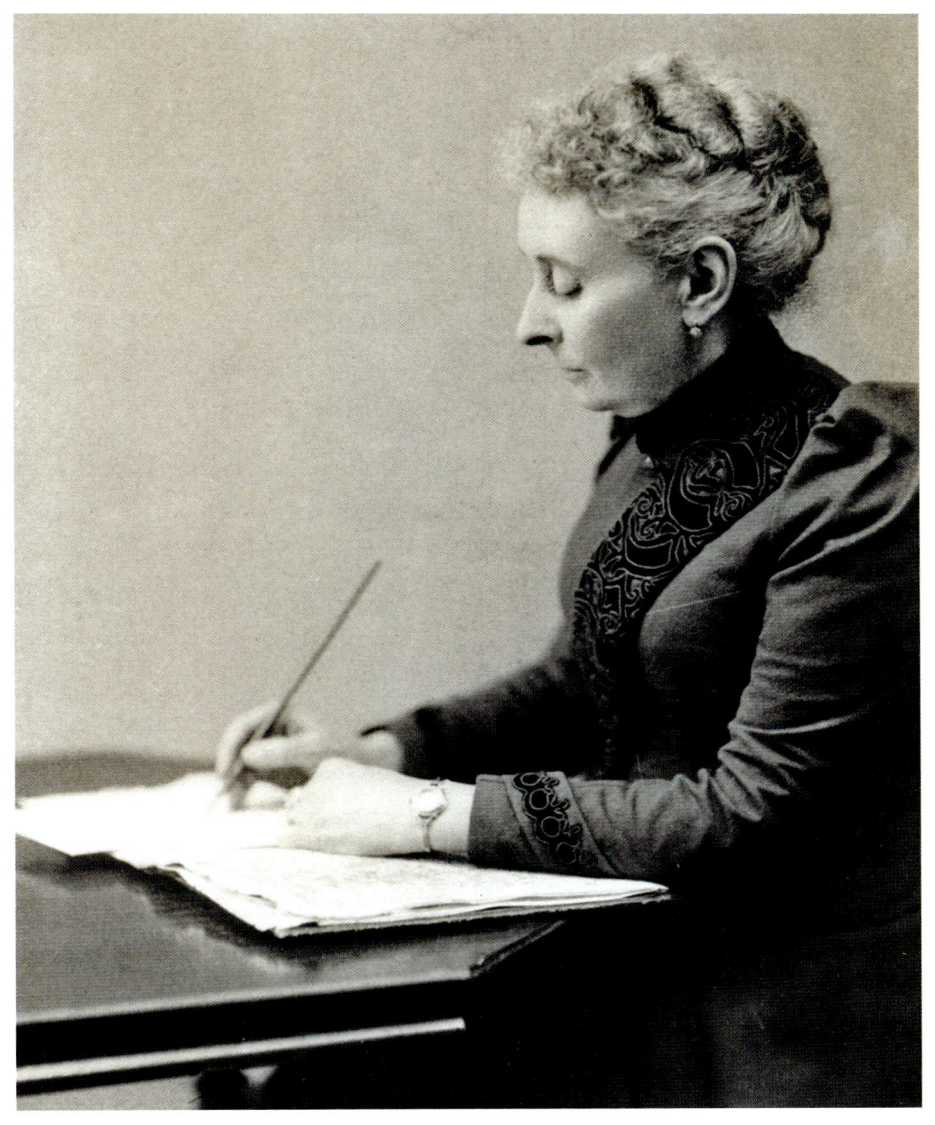

Mary Langdon Down.
© Langdon Down Museum of Learning Disability/London Metropolitan Archive

The whole of this major undertaking at Normansfield, which had two hundred patients at one point, was overseen on a day-to-day basis for over thirty years by Dr John Langdon-Down's wife, Mary. Her care for her patients can be seen in the large collection of letters she wrote to the relatives.[29] A truly remarkable woman.

Dr John himself, whilst the Superintendent and the force behind Normansfield, was still working at the London Hospital, had a successful private practice at 81 Harley Street and wrote extensive medical papers. He died a rich man – leaving over £20,000 in his will, a value which in current times would be between £2 million and £22 million, depending on which system of calculation is used.[30] The term 'mongol' or 'mongoloid' which he had coined was used by doctors as a medical classification until after the Second World War – long after the original thinking behind the name had been superseded. Only in the early 1960s, when there was a move to replace what was thought to have become an insensitive as well as a completely inaccurate term, did the question arise of what such people should be called. It was agreed by nearly all the experts that it should become 'Down's syndrome' in memory of Dr John Langdon-Down and his two sons Reginald and Percival, who had done such constructive and caring work in this field for a hundred years.

However, there were important differences between the two organizations. First, Normansfield had only a very small farm. Secondly, quite a high proportion of the patients or residents were only at Normansfield for a relatively short period of time. (40% were there for less than two years according to the U3A study).[31] Thirdly, patients at the new Farm Colony were to be relatively able-bodied and not too severely mentally retarded. And fourthly, the Princess Christian Farm Colony never had children, although at one time there were plans for them.

So, in spite of the differences, there are obvious connections and parallels between Normansfield and the Farm Colony. Normansfield had been started forty years before the Hildenborough project and Dr Reginald Langdon-Down had, as we have seen, worked at Normansfield with his father for over ten years before he took charge at the Farm Colony. Clearly what he had learnt from those years was brought to his work at Princess Christian; and the prime motivation behind both organizations was the same. There are also parallels between what happened to the two organizations at the end of the twentieth century. Normansfield continued as a charity until 1951 when it became an NHS hospital; and members of the Langdon-Down family, firstly Dr Percival and then followed by his son, Norman, were active in the organization from 1900 until 1970. After a difficult period in the 1970s, Normansfield recovered but, as with Princess Christian, it started to be wound up in the late 1980s, finally closing in 1997. This then was the hospital on which Princess Christian's Farm Colony was to be based.[32]

Langdon-Down Family Tree, compiled by Joyce Field.

Joseph Almond Down
b: 7 Mar 1783 London
d: 1853 St Germans, Cornwall

Hannah Haydon
m: 7 May 1808 St George, Hanover Square, London

John Langdon Haydon Down
b: 1828 Torpoint, Cornwall, England
d: 1896 Teddington, Middlesex

Mary Crellin
b: about 1829 St George in the East, London, England
m: 1860 Hackney
d: 1900 Kingston, Surrey

Percival Langdon-Down
b: 1868 Kingston
d: 19 Aug 1925 Kingston

Helena Augusta Marguerite Bigwood
m: 1899 Brentford, Middlesex, England
d: 1957

Barbara Langdon-Down
b: 7 Feb 1909 Kingston
d: 1995 Buckinghamshire

Sydney Charles Thomas Littlewood
m: 1934 Staines, Middlesex
d: 1967

Norman Langdon-Down
b: 1905 Kingston
d: 1991 Surrey

Mary Langdon-Down
b: 1902 Kingston

Edward T Cooper
m: 1927 Kingston, Surrey

Reginald Langdon-Down
b: 1866 Reigate, Surrey, England
d: 1955 Middlesex

Jane Jarvie Cleveland
b: 1864 Umballa, India
m: 1895 Marylebone, Middlesex, England
d: 1917 Kingston, Surrey

Amy Ruth Turnbull MBE
b: about 1878 Shanghai, China
m: 1922 Hildenborough, Kent
d: 24 Jan 1942 Teddington, Middlesex

Antony Turnbull Langdon-Down
b: 1923 Kingston, Surrey
d: 2010

Sylvia Wiles
m: 1947 Wycombe, Bucks
d: 2007

Jill E Caruth
m: 1954 Marylebone, Middlesex, England
d: 2001

John Cleveland Langdon-Down
b: 1905 Marylebone, Middlesex, England
d: 1970 Richmond-upon-Thames

Elspie Langdon-Down
b: 1899 Teddington, Middlesex, England
d: 1987 North Dorset

Archibald R Cusden
m: 1933 Kingston

Stella Langdon-Down
b: 1896 Marylebone, Middlesex, England

Walter Russell Brain
b: 23 Oct 1895 Reading, Berkshire
m: 1920 Kingston, Surrey
b: 29 Dec 1966 Kingston, Surrey

The First Staff and 'Colonists'

In spite of the uncertainty about when exactly the Hildenborough plans were first discussed; when the initial land was purchased; and when the first buildings were erected and converted – let alone exactly when the first boy/male 'colonists' arrived – it seems that sometime around 1905 and 1907 that the main buildings were built and existing buildings adapted.

The main new building was drawn out in 1904 and became known as the Oast House. It was designed by the architects, Bertram Clough Williams-Ellis (who later became well known for designing and building the village of Portmeirion in North Wales and who was eventually knighted) with his then partner, James Scott. It aimed to incorporate local building styles within the general Arts and Crafts movement and it seems possible that the Williams-Ellis design was inspired by an existing oast house. As can be seen from the wording on the architects' drawings which follow (page 28), it was to hold twenty-five feeble-minded boys, a master and a matron. It had a reasonable sized bathroom by the standards of its day, although the twenty-five beds were fitted into the dormitory of under fifty foot by fifteen foot.[33] The new building had a double oast at one end which led into the main living quarters, with a single oast at the far end.

A report in the Kent & Sussex Courier (19 November 1908) describes a fire in the new Colony and mentions that there were twenty 'protégés or colonists' in this initial period. There was a further fire in 1909 and another in 1914 – although the last was only a small incident of fat catching fire in the kitchen. Nevertheless, the local Fire Brigade must have felt they were beginning to know the early Colony well.

By 1909, if not earlier, Dr Reginald Langdon-Down seems to have acquired a nearby house, 'Oaklands', in Vines Lane, Hildenborough from Lord Derby's estate,[34] although in the 1911 census Dr Reginald, his wife and son, John, are still shown at Normansfield, with their two daughters, Stella and Elspie, away at school.

Oaklands was a large, attractive house with generous proportions built around 1860 of Kentish ragstone and situated in open countryside. It was a hundred yards from the Farm and around two hundred yards from the main Princess Christian buildings, so a convenient place for the Langdon-Downs to have as a base. However, Reginald continued to be the joint Medical Superintendent of Normansfield with his brother, Percival, from the turn of the century until Percival's death in 1925, when Helen, Percival's widow, joined Reginald in charge of Normansfield. Seemingly,

From the Start of an Idea to The Second World War

Reginald continued to play an active role at Normansfield until after World War II when he would have been in his late seventies. At that point his nephew, Norman, became the Medical Superintendent at Normansfield. By the end of the War, Reginald would have been in charge of Normansfield for around fifty years and, for a good part of the time, he had his own private practice in Welbeck Street, London. With these tasks in mind, it is not clear how much time he would have been able to spend at Oaklands doing work on Princess Christian affairs. Perhaps his supervision of the Farm Colony was the kind of role the chairman of a firm would have today – overseeing board meetings, appointing senior staff, reading and commenting on reports of progress and suggesting ideas based on his own experience, but not necessarily living very much at Oaklands. With the return journey to and from Normansfield around ninety miles by car, involving a three hour drive each way, Oaklands would have been a useful overnight home for maybe three or four nights a month but perhaps not a fully fledged family home.[35]

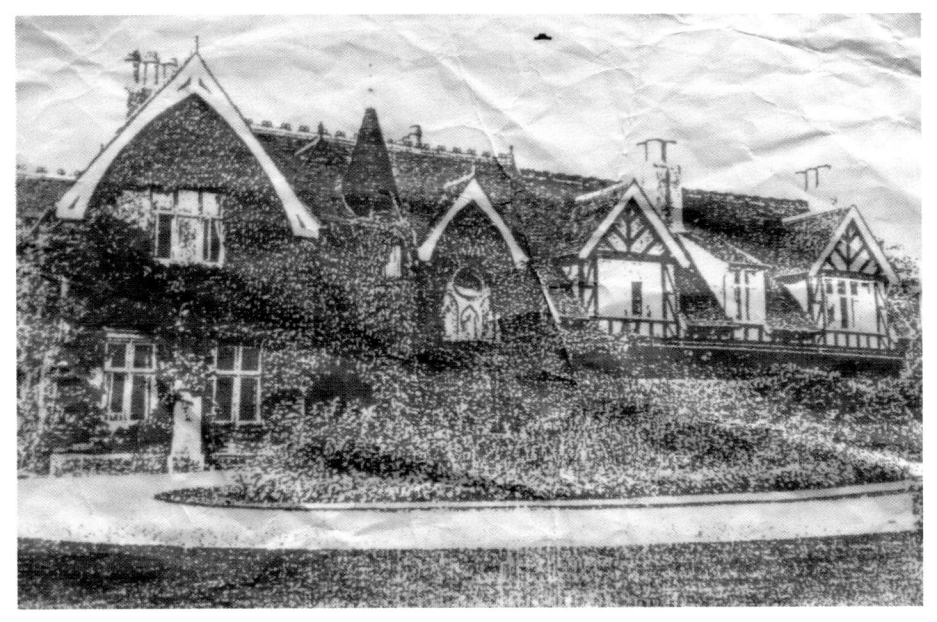

Oaklands – later renamed Alexander House – at the beginning of the 20th century.

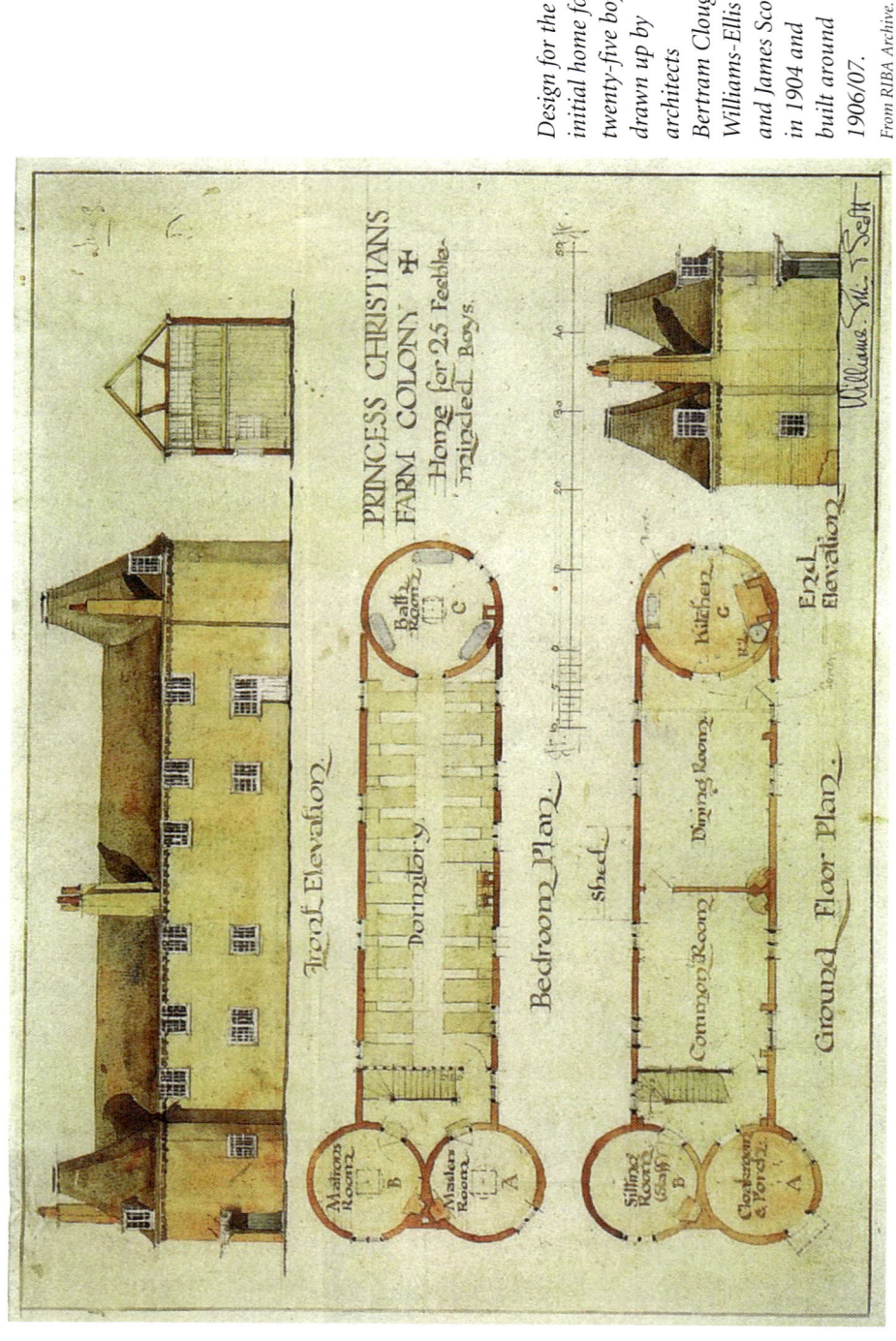

Design for the initial home for twenty-five boys drawn up by architects Bertram Clough Williams-Ellis and James Scott in 1904 and built around 1906/07.
From RIBA Archive.

From the Start of an Idea to The Second World War

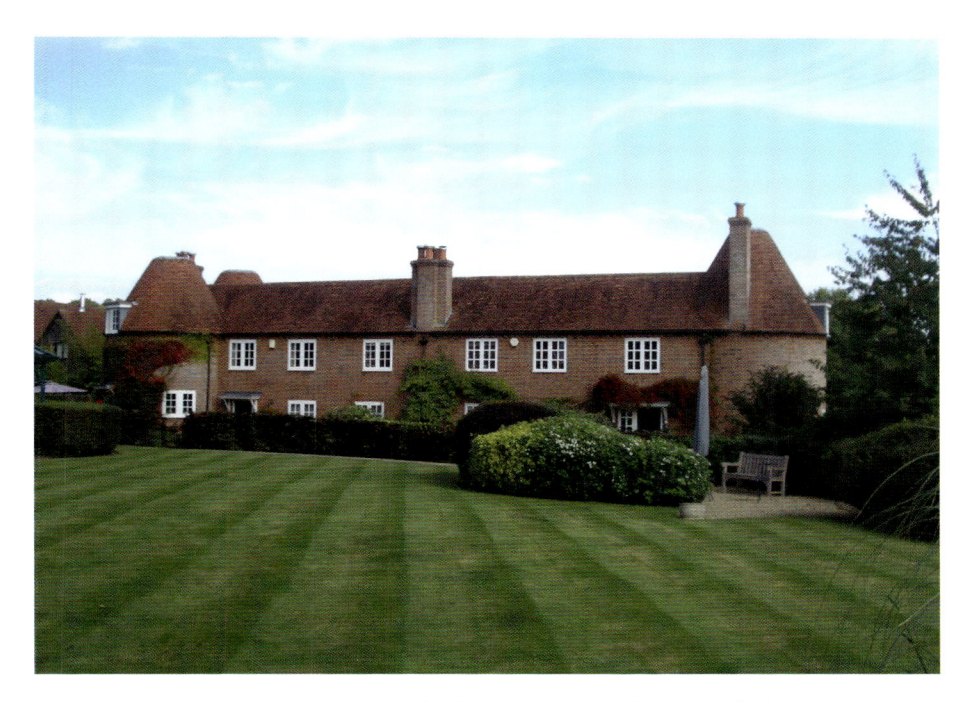

The present Oast House which was rebuilt in 2001 using the original plans.
Photos: Anna Rowley

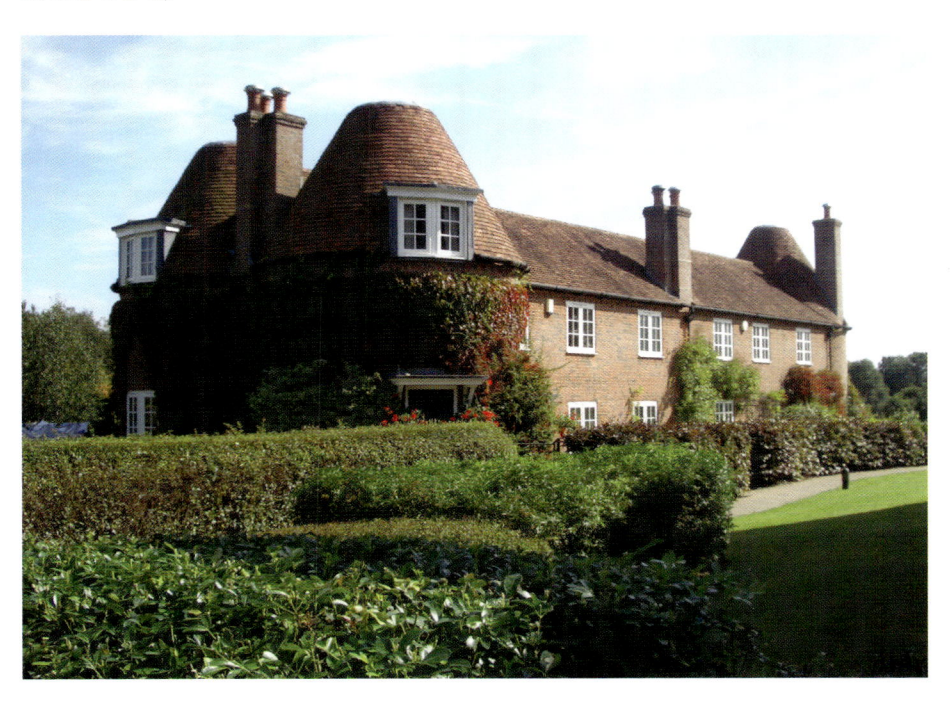

The Architect at the Princess Christian Farm Colony

Sir Bertram Clough Williams-Ellis CBE MC 1883-1978 designed two of the principal buildings at the Farm Colony – the first, when he was only twenty. (However, it was not unheard of for very young architects to be given commissions. William Harvey was also twenty when he was given the huge task of designing the Bournville Model Village in 1895).

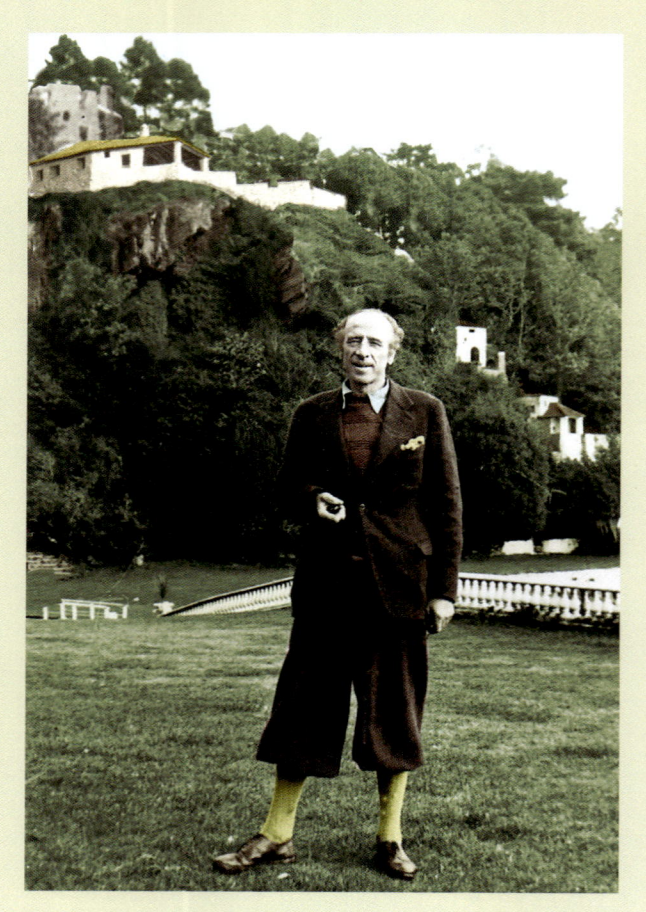

Bertram Clough Williams Ellis ca 1928 aged around 45 at the village he designed at Portmeirion, N.W. Wales
© Portmeirion Ltd

Although born in England, Williams-Ellis moved back to the family estate, Plas Brondanw, in North Wales when young and for the rest of his life continued to devote a good deal of time beautifying it. (The estate is nowadays open to the public).

He had been to Oundle School and then on to Trinity College, Cambridge to read Natural Sciences. However, he did not take his degree and instead decided to become an architect. In 1903/04 he started studying at the Architectural Association (which he found by looking in the London telephone directory) but left after a short time. Nevertheless, he set up his own architectural practice with a friend, James Scott.

One of their earlier commissions around 1903/04 was for the main boys' house at the Princess Christian Farm Colony in Hildenborough, Kent. He became involved in the Cheap Cottage Movement and designed cottages for labourers near his family estate using local materials – stone, slate and roughcast. In 1905 he was designing pairs of cottages to be sold at £316. Later he won a competition where he designed cottages for Merrow Down in Surrey for £110. In 1915/16, working by himself, he designed the Girls' Home at Princess Christian. (It later became known as Glen House). In the 1920s he designed a few individual buildings and his major work, the village of Portmeirion on the North West coast of Wales.

He also wrote a book about his experiments with ancient building methods including using compressed earth, cob, pisé, chalk and clay. His architectural output was not large but he became famous and was knighted more for his writing and enthusiasm about the environment, where he became 'The Grand Old Man' of architecture and conservation, concerned about creeping urbanization and the need to preserve fine buildings. He was an early supporter of the National Trust and his aim was to build and encourage classically styled buildings which fitted harmoniously within the landscape – something which he achieved both at Portmeirion and at the Princess Christian Farm Colony.

Sources: various, including Wikipedia and http://letchworthgardencity.com/heritage

Very ironically (and sadly), Dr Reginald and his family had a personal reason for being involved with Mongolism/Down's syndrome children, apart from his own and his father's work on the subject. Although it was not widely mentioned or known at the time, his third child, Jack (John Cleveland Langdon-Down), born in 1905 when his wife, Jane, was forty-one, suffered from the condition. Jane apparently never really came to terms what she felt was a misfortune but Jack grew up and became a well-loved member of the family, living a happy life and dying in 1970 at Normansfield aged sixty-five. (The 1911 census which, as we have seen, showed John with his parents at Normansfield, does not mark John as 'feeble-minded' in the relevant column. Perhaps his parents were shy of mentioning that one of their own children had a problem when they were running a hospital for people with a similar disability.)

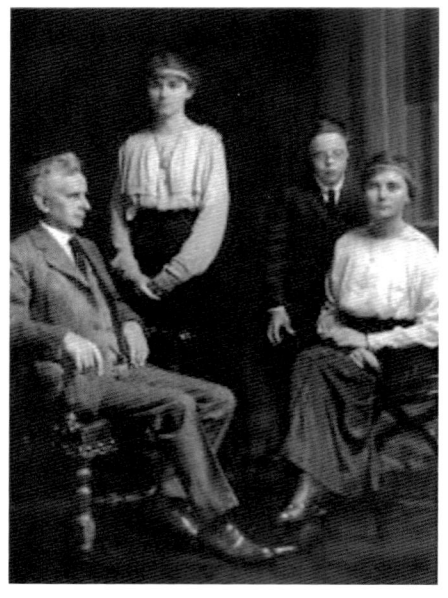

Family of Reginald Langdon Down from around 1913. Left to right Reginald, daughters Stella and Elspie and son, John
© Langdon Down Museum of Learning Disability

The National Association or some sub-committee under Doctor Reginald is said in some local notes to have bought the farm or the two farms in 1908.[36] However, as we have seen, there must have been discussions, if not formal agreement, somewhat earlier. New Trench Farm was described when it was bought for £5,000[37] from Lord Derby's estate as "a bijou house with farm premises."[38] It consisted of the main farm house and farm buildings; an oast house and two labourers cottages. Upper Hollenden Farm – whenever it was bought – had fewer buildings, a farm house and several outbuildings. In all the farm land was about a hundred and twenty acres. We have a reasonable idea of the layout of the two farms from the 1900 map shown at the end of this chapter. (The building on the SE corner of New Trench Farm appears to have a double oast house and the new main building for the men, based on the theme of a Kent oast house, would have been built roughly on this site.)

For the first four or five years the Farm Colony purposely concentrated on "lads between sixteen and twenty three." From the beginning it was intended that the Farm would help towards the Colony being self-supporting. Before too long, there were cows and poultry, and the growing of vegetables, all of which were intended to create income as well as to help feed the Colony. In 1910 Lady Frederick Brudenell-Bruce, a supporter who had been on a visit to the Farm Colony, described how the Boys' Home was doing excellent work. She had seen them planting potatoes, "a really good and useful crop being put into the ground. The boys also did carpentering &c."[40] So, although parents or the authorities who were responsible for the individual 'boys' were normally expected to pay for the running costs (sometimes according to their means), a small proportion of the costs would have been offset by what the Colony produced itself. As the Colony developed, it expanded into a fully working farm with a pig breeding unit and a dairy herd with its own milking parlour. A bull was kept so that the herd could be increased in size and part of the 120 acres was used for producing hay and straw for the cattle. This meant that horses had to be kept to undertake such tasks as the ploughing, harrowing and reseeding. Even in the 1940s, two local residents, Bill Richardson and Ron Wood, remember the remaining horse pulling a cart full of dung down Riding Lane to be left in piles down the fields for the 'boys' in their ex-Army clothes to spread out. "Actually we called it the 'shit cart' but perhaps you don't say that in public," says Bill. Another resident remembers the 'boys' in the field, standing by the large piles of dung, enjoying themselves by throwing the dung up in the air and getting covered in it – with much laughter. He thought the Colony must have been relieved by this time to have its own laundry. A milk round had been started early in the establishment of the Colony, first on foot and then with a pony and milk float. This local service continued until 1935 and was resumed after the War.

The 'boys' were not only taught about farming. As we have heard, they were taught carpentry from an early date and the Colony took orders for "hen houses, hen coops, potting sheds etc.," making a reasonable profit on the sales. They were also taught bricklaying. By 1921/22, we have a fuller description of the 'boys' work from the long-serving, highly regarded Superintendent, Miss Pitman.[41] Her report is given later but it confirms that a wide variety of work was taught to the 'boys', almost certainly from the beginning of the Colony. We also know that from the start of the Colony the 'boys' regularly participated in religious services somewhere in the farm buildings which were conducted by the vicar from Hildenborough. In 1912 the Hildenborough Vestry Minutes[42] noted that "regular services had been held at the Princess Christian Farm Colony and they were very nice services indeed, the 110 inmates joining heartily in the singing, and often proving by their display of knowledge that they were not so void of understanding as they were supposed to be." It is interesting and somewhat ironic to contrast this positive view of the 'colonists' with the more lurid views expressed by some of those appealing for funds, who clearly thought that by frightening local people about the dangerousness of 'the feeble-minded', more money could be raised to help keep the feeble-minded away from ordinary people. For example, one of those trying to raise money, Mrs Pearce Clark from The Drive, Sevenoaks, wrote, "It can hardly be necessary to say much about the urgent need there is to segregate the feeble-minded. For just as the inheritance of ability has been proved, so the inheritance of weakness and depravity is no less certain."[43] More quotes from the Colony's supporters are given later when the problems of raising funds are described. Only as few were what today we would consider sympathetic or constructive.

The 1911 Census

The 1911 census returns relating to the Farm Colony give fuller details of how the expansion was continuing. The Superintendent, or Lady Superintendent as she was sometimes called, was Mrs Jeannie Fry, although the Christian name is not clear on the census form. She was forty-four and lived in 'Colony Cottage', a house which had six rooms. Other staff were William Edwin Tull and his wife, Sarah, both thirty-nine, who were called House Master and House Matron respectively. They lived in the Main House. The number of rooms is given as eleven. It was also occupied by an Assistant Master, Charles Alexander Rooke aged thirty, who seems to have been concerned with supervising the work on the Farm. This building was presumably the original farm house. It had twenty-five male residents. The Clough Williams-Ellis building, the Oast House, where the number of rooms is given as six, was holding its full complement of twenty-four residents as well as two staff, William Coles Seagrave, whose occupation is described as 'House and Garden' and his wife Alice, whose occupation is described as 'Dairy and House'. (When describing an institution, the census gave the number of rooms which included the kitchen – but not the scullery, landing, lobby, closet, bathroom or office.) So, taken overall, the census shows that by 1911 the number of 'colonists' had expanded from the original twenty to forty-nine, all males. The photo of the relevant census page for the Colony (Appendix 3) gives full details but the ages were largely between seventeen and twenty-one, although there was one aged fourteen and two aged twenty-seven.

The census could indicate the staff:colonist ratio was 1:8, with the forty-nine 'colonists' and six staff. However, additional local men were almost certainly employed on the Farm to show the 'colonists' what to do and to keep an eye on them, as well as further staff to train the 'boys' in the other skills such as carpentry and building. There could also have been a few local women who may have helped with overseeing such things as the cooking, although we have no details of who they were or how many there were. In any case, for the most part the 'colonists' were expected to look after themselves, doing their own cleaning and clothes washing as well as cooking for themselves.

The census has a last column headed 'infirmity'. The census notes tell the enumerator to record details of any person who is totally deaf, deaf and dumb, totally blind, lunatic, imbecile or feeble-minded, together with the age at which he or she became afflicted. In the case of Princess Christian, the enumerator has put 'feeble-minded' at the top of the relevant pages followed by a long list of ditto marks. So there is no information about whether the 'colonists' had been born with their infirmity or how severe their problems were. However, it is worth noting that in 1911 and indeed for the next eighty years, the 'colonists' or patients or residents had a variety of conditions which had to be helped.[44] Looking at the places of birth, few came from local towns or villages; and only four were born in Kent – in Tunbridge Wells, Dover, Bromley and Orpington. The Colony was, therefore, definitely not intended to be a local facility and in the next seventy to eighty years only a few local people lived at the Colony, or the Hospital as it became.

The Formal Opening Planned for 1910 and Further Developments

From various newspaper articles and letters in the newspapers, mainly written by Trustees of the National Association, it is clear that a large formal opening ceremony with Princess Christian present was planned for 3 June 1910. Unfortunately, King Edward VII, the Princess's uncle, was inconsiderate enough to die in May and with heavy mourning resulting, so the Farm Colony ceremony had to be postponed. The formal start of the Colony, however, still seemed to be regarded as 1910, even if the actual ceremony did not happen until the following summer and even if the Farm Colony had already had young men living and working there for two or three years. In the period leading up to what was going to be the formal opening in June 1910, the National Association must have decided to have a fund-raising drive locally. The newspapers in Sevenoaks and Tonbridge had lengthy letters and articles about meetings, particularly to request funds. One letter in particular is worth quoting because it expresses views which are so different to what we feel today about the 'feeble-minded'.[45]

"Sir – Every year newspapers team with figures demonstrating the increase of feeblemindedness and lunacy, and the crimes resulting from these causes; yet the public look on at this rising flood of degeneracy without attempting to avert it. 'If there is a positive increase in the numbers of feebleminded and lunatics,' says Professor Clifford Allbutt, 'it is because we are doing our best to breed them… Feeblemindedness is largely hereditary and it is therefore one of the most preventable disease.'" The letter goes on to give a reasonably accurate and sympathetic description of the work already being done at the Farm Colony and to appeal for money both to pay off debts already incurred and to go towards new facilities for young girls "who are in greater danger than all others." After more practicalities, the tune reverts to its earlier theme: "a medical specialist has said 'more Nations have sunk to utter insignificance as the result of moral, intellectual and physical degeneracy than by war, famine or any other condition.'"

Another letter to the newspaper also gives an indication of the scale of the Farm Colony's debts: "... So far the National Association has raised £4,300 but another £8,000 is yet required to clear off the debt for the land purchased; to build more homes (including for young girls) and to establish a school and homes for feebleminded children of both sexes."[46]

Strangely, the same newspaper – on the same day and the same page – had another letter about the Farm Colony, this time from the local lady, Mrs Lylie Pearce Clark, from whom we have heard before. On this occasion, she is much less alarmist than in her earlier letter. She says that, as the State gives no help, "the care of this particular class falls entirely on the voluntary agencies now at work. Where we come across the feeble-minded in our Workhouses or in their own homes, we cannot but be struck by their apathetic, and often miserable appearance. In the Boys Home, already started at the Colony …. they are trained …. and, in their own dim way, they realize that they are of some use and are therefore made happy." She then goes on to ask for more funds – perhaps a more appealing approach than the one mentioned above by the Association's representative? But perhaps before coming to the view that Mrs Clark was a caring and humane middle-class/upper-class lady, we should remember that she was the lady who had sent the letter, quoted earlier, that implied the feeble-minded had to be segregated to prevent them breeding.

Six weeks later, at the end of April 1910, the fund raising was continuing, this time with the aim of getting the great and the good together – or as many as they could, because it seems a good number of the local titled ladies and gentlemen sent their apologies.[47] The meeting was convened by the Lord Bishop of Rochester and was held at the Bishop's Court in Sevenoaks. Sir William Chance who was in the Chair on behalf of the National Association gave the address. After his plea for more funds, various other local dignitaries gave their reasons why the Farm Colony needed help, including an unnamed doctor who plainly specialized in helping the feeble-minded. Unless they were supported, he said "they end up in prison – not because they are criminal but because they had not sufficient strength of mind to resist committing some criminal acts." Others present said that workhouses, too, contained many who were feeble-minded. Thirty pounds was collected at this particular meeting but it is not known how much money was raised by this campaign overall. However, expansion was still continuing. By 1910, a farm house, perhaps at Upper Hollenden Farm, had been converted to hold twenty-two boys and by July 1914 the Colony had about a hundred boys according to a local newspaper. In February 1915, the Association auctioned off twenty acres of 'underwood'. Perhaps it was to help pay towards the next major project.

The Girls' Home and the Arrival of Female 'Colonists' 1916/17

The new expansion was to build accommodation for younger women. Once again, they were to be chosen by the overarching organization – the National Association. While the majority of the 'girls' chosen would have had some real 'learning disability' – as it was to become named seventy years later – there would have certainly been a proportion who were inconvenient to their parents or an embarrassment. Embarrassment included being pregnant and single. The Mental Deficiency Act 1913 – for which the National Association had fought – included a clause which allowed local authorities to put unmarried mothers who were deemed defective into a mental institution or a workhouse.[48] This certainly happened at the Farm Colony because in the 1950s and 1960s, there were elderly ladies who had come to Princess Christian for just that reason. However, there are no records of why or how men or women were judged suitable to be at the

Farm Colony. At this point, it is worth explaining what has repeatedly been mentioned by those who have been concerned with the Colony or just those who lived locally. The male 'colonists' were always referred to as the 'boys' even if twenty or thirty years after their arrival they had become forty, fifty or even sixty. Similarly, the women of whatever age were always referred to as the 'girls'. There had been at least some 'girls' at the Colony before the First World War. Although there had been none in the 1911 census, newspaper reports in the summer of 1912 mention women working usefully at the Colony with their own staff to look after them.

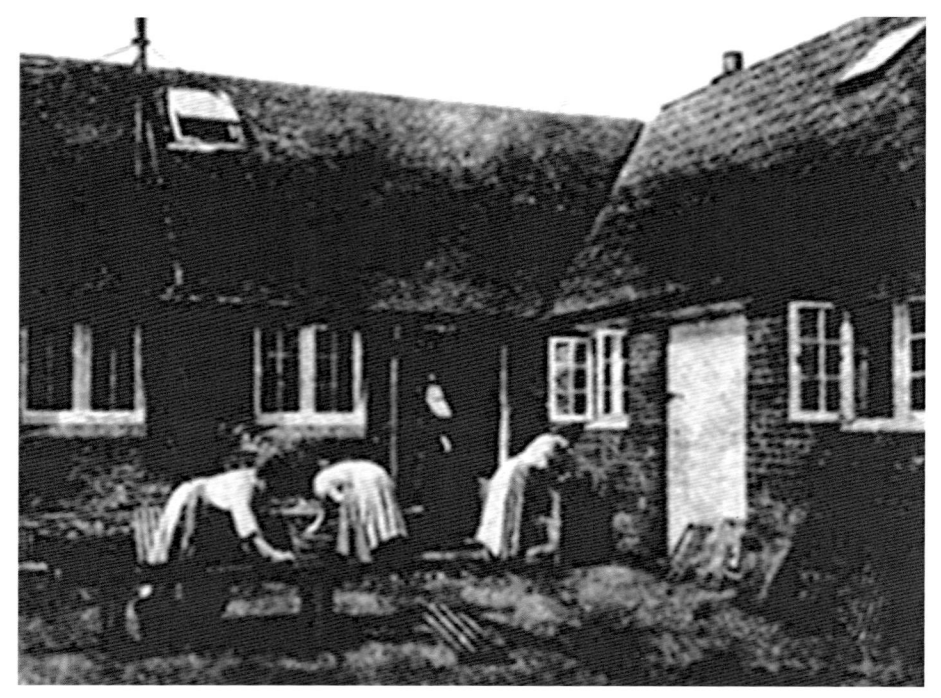

Some of the 'girls' at work, Summer 1912
Photo: Sevenoaks Chronicle & Kentish Advertiser 7 June 1912

However, the major Princess Christian expansion, which had been discussed by the National Association since at least 1910, came to fruition in 1916 when a large home for female residents was built half a mile up the main drive through New Trench Farm. It was referred to as the Girls' Home. (It was not called 'Glen House' until around 1960, as we will see later.) Bearing in mind this expansion was carried out when the First World War was in one of its most difficult years, with shortages of manpower and resources, it must have been quite an undertaking. Additionally, its architect, once again Clough Williams-Ellis, was away in the War with the Welsh Guards earning his M.C. We know more about the architecture of this building than any other part of the Colony because the plans and elevations are kept by RIBA[49] and, even more so, because much later it became a Grade II listed building. So a good deal was written about it. There seems to have been some connection between the two Langdon-Down sons and Williams-Ellis. They were all at Trinity College, Cambridge, although the Langdon-Downs were there around fifteen years earlier. But however they knew each other, the new Girls' Home was larger and much grander than the original 'boys' house oast. As the plans show, it was to have twenty-five 'girls' on the east side and twenty five 'girls' on the identical west side. The facilities were on a more civilized scale than the 'boys' home, with workrooms and lavatories downstairs; and, the location, surrounded by fields on all sides was beautiful – as well as being a good way from the 'boys'!

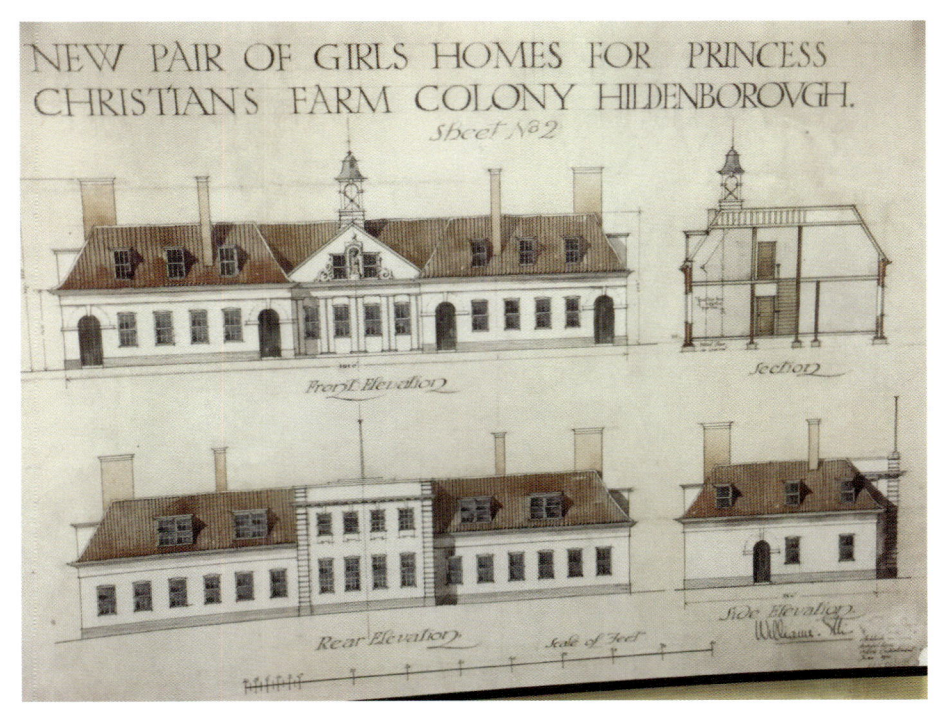

above and following page
Plans and Elevations of the Girls' Home (later Glen House) dated June 1916.
From RIBA Archive

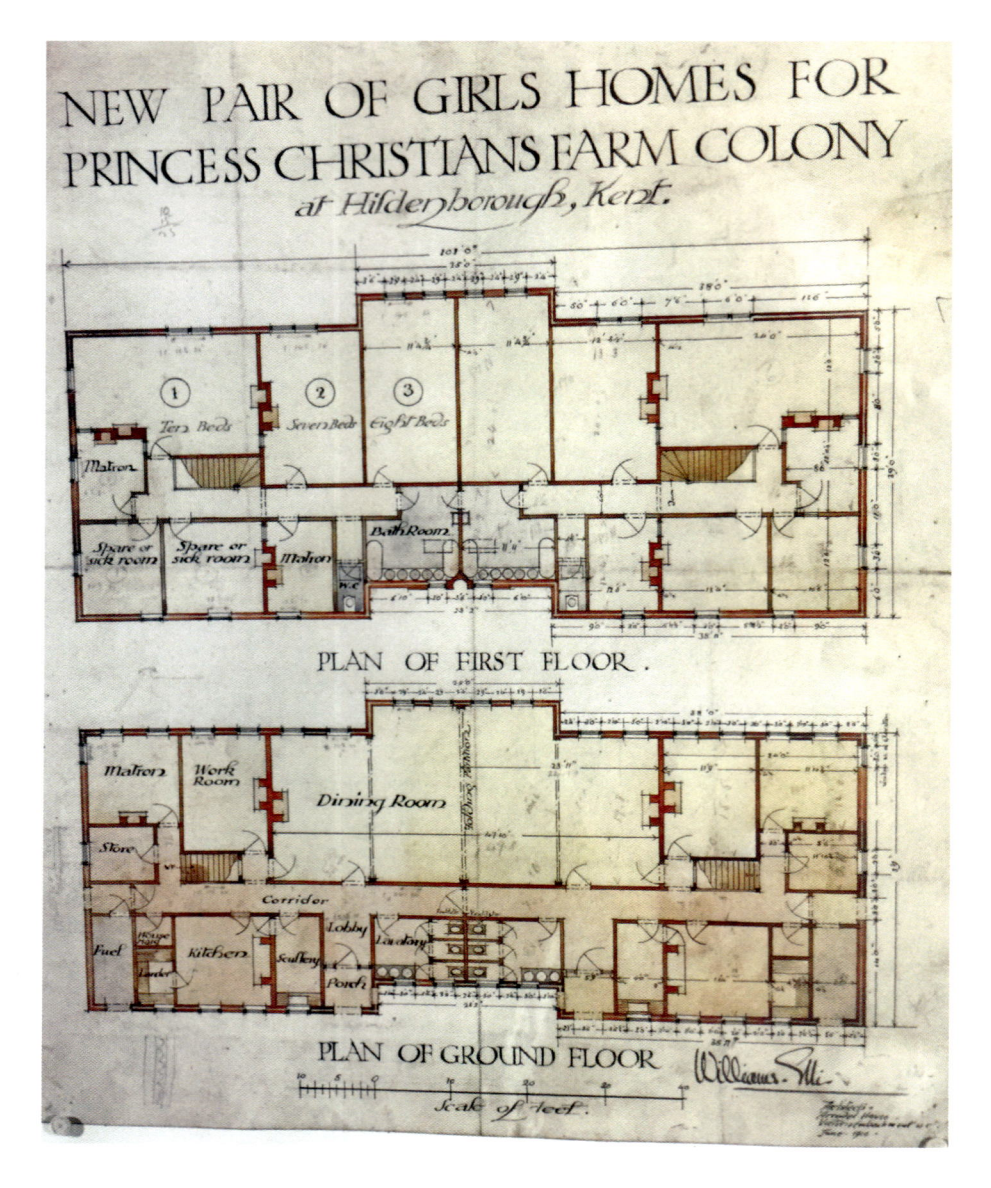

The Princess Christian Farm Colony and Hospital 1895–1995

In 1923, alterations and the addition of an extension on the north side of the Girls' Home were made under architects, Conrad Birdwood Willcocks; and at some point in the early 1930s, there were further additions when it was said that the 'boys' from the Colony helped with the work. We know that the 'boys' were still being trained to be relatively competent in both bricklaying and carpentry, because special prizes were given for both trades in July 1926.[50]

The training or the occupations of the young women who were to live in the Girls' Home were clearly indicated by the five foot statue that Williams-Ellis designed to go into a large niche above the main door. From a distance it could well be a Madonna. However, rather than a statue with religious significance, it is a representation of what the 'girls' in the new Girls' Home should aspire to be – a well-balanced domestic servant. The statue shows a youngish girl with a cotton cap, a long dress and an apron.

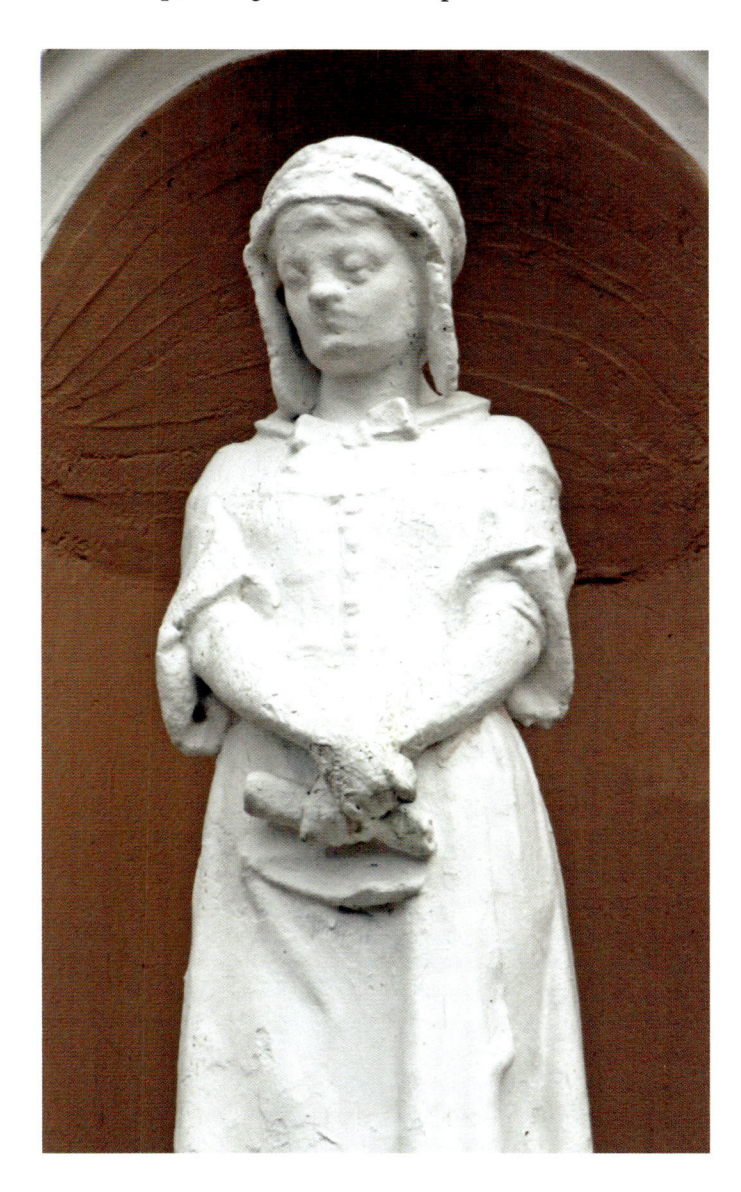

1916 Statue above main door at the Girls' Home representing the girls living in the home.
Photo: Charles Linton/ Juliet Rowley

Clough Williams-Ellis had also included a small bell tower as a central feature above the main door and the statue. One assumes that there was a bell with a bell-rope used by the staff to summon the residents to meals or to start their various jobs (although no signs of the bell itself or its mechanism for ringing it remained in 2000).

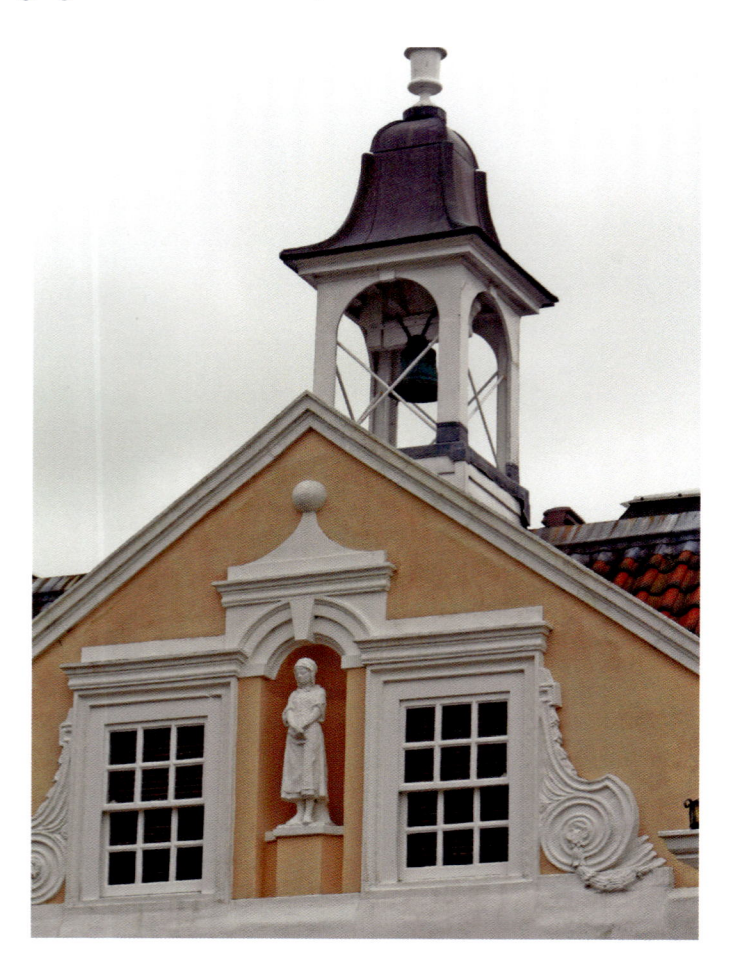

The Bell Tower at Girls' Home in 2015.
Photo: Charles Linton/Juliet Rowley

From the beginning, the milk round had been one of the most profitable parts of Princess Christian's income and the 'girls' became part of the team. Concrete proof of the pony or ponies used to pull the milk float around the district was found in 2015 by local resident, Pat Davies. On the bank of the Hilden Brook at a place which must have been the Colony's rubbish dump (there were no rubbish collections in those days), he came upon a fair number of small, worn horse shoes.

The 'girls' also did the laundry for the main Colony, using wooden wash tubs for 'coppers'. (Once a year the tubs were also used for cooking the Christmas puddings.) Flat irons, heated on special coke stoves, were used to do the ironing. And just as the 'boys' were taught to do a variety of jobs, the 'girls' were taught a range of work, including sewing (Miss Weeks was the sewing mistress in 1923), cooking and cleaning; and some at least would certainly have helped with the preparation of the meals for the Colony as a whole. Although we do not know the details about the early days, the various jobs would have been allocated to the 'girls' on the basis of their individual ability – which would have varied quite considerably when one looks at later papers about the Farm Colony. As well as training for work related jobs, it is clear that the 'girls' also had lessons in crafts. There are mentions of raffia work and coir mats made by the 'girls' in newspaper reports of summer fêtes – and folk dancing, singing and small plays, including Peter Pan in 1927 which seems to have been relatively complex, were performed at various open days. The 1921/22 Annual Report does not give any details of the work done by the 'girls' which it says "goes on steadily under the same female officers", in contrast to the 'boys', where the House Attendant has been sacked for "lacking a sense of responsibility." However, the Annual Report does add that the female officers "are very interested in the individual training of the girls in their various departments." At one stage, the 'girls' must have made or helped make mattresses because in 1937 there is a newspaper article which praises them for giving the finished products to the poor. The work and the training – particularly for the less handicapped 'girls' – would not have been very different to that given to women in the better contemporary lunatic asylums and workhouses. Indeed, it was not dissimilar to that provided in local schools at this time. So these skills were not in any way demeaning to the residents – the 'girls'.

Work for the 'Boys' in the 1920s

The 1921/22 Annual Report is more forthcoming about the work done by the 'boys'. In a section written by the Superintendent – presumably the renowned Miss Pitman, although she is not named – it reports that one group of 'boys' continued to be taught about gardening. Another group, which had been increasing in number, had been working on the farm. "They are very interested in their cattle and in growing crops. In addition, our piggeries have been an unfailing source of pleasure to both boys and girls with the arrival of seven litters within a few weeks of each other. Still more are to follow! The carpenter and his boys have been fully occupied throughout the year, and all over the Colony the results of their work can be seen. Pig shelters have been made, wire fencing put up, a coal store for the Girls' Home built, and painting, repairing and general redecoration of all buildings carried out. The annexe at the Oast House has been match-boarded and a covered way erected between the main building and the Oast House. Additionally, a cottage was converted by the estate carpenters with help from the 'boys'. The upper storey roof was raised and it was redecorated, so that five 'boys' could live there." We know from other descriptions that the re-done building, which must have been on the New Trench Farm site, had a "fine hung tiling on the upper storey… which became known as The Hostel". It had a large garden at the side which was used for growing vegetables, as well as having several well-tended herbaceous borders at the front. Miss Pitman goes on to mention the expansion of the mat-making department. "One lad who cannot speak and has always worked in the garden, installed himself in front of a mat-making frame and insisted on being taught. He has proved himself to be one of the best workers in this department … Excellent work has again been accomplished in the boot shop, both in repairs and new work." She goes on to praise "the garden boys". So clearly, there was a range of jobs which were done, in addition to the work on the Farm and the building and carpentry. We have the name of carpentry teacher in 1927, Francis Lones – although, sadly, we only know of him because the local paper reported his suicide.

The Superintendent's report for the AGM goes on to list what was done under the heading 'Recreation'. "Drill has been continued daily throughout the year. The boys are developing a keen interest in football and cricket, and the swings are a favourite. In addition to organized walks, picnics and concerts, parties of boys or girls ['boys' would have gone separately from 'girls'] are taken to the local cinema when suitable films are exhibited. This gives special pleasure and provides a topic of conversation for days afterwards".

Choosing the Farm 'Colonists' in the early 1920s

There are no details of how the National Association chose the men and women who came to the Princess Christian Farm Colony in the early years but quite clearly age and their particular learning disability were major factors. Initially, as we have seen, the age had been around eighteen to early twenties and they would have to be within the definition of 'feeble-minded'. One guesses that finance also played a part. Was there sufficient funding for that particular person? A few residents probably came from Normansfield. From early 1920s documents we know that the National Association had a waiting list. (They had 445 applications in 1921/22.) So the Association would have to have chosen carefully those whom they would send to the Colony.[51] We read that some of the applicants would go to other houses run by the Association; some were advised to stay with their parents; and it seems that a few ended up in the 'real', public lunatic asylums.[52] However, throughout all its life, only those whose physical and mental capacity would enable them to work at the Colony Farm, would be sent there. In the 1921/22 Annual Report twenty-one men were admitted and fifteen discharged (one further 'boy' died) out of a total of one hundred and forty-one 'colonists' (seventy-three males and sixty-eight females). Of the fifteen discharged, three went to mental hospitals, two went home and one went to one of the National Association's Approved Houses. Of the eight females discharged, five went back to their parents, one went into service, with another going to a Training Home for servants and the last – presumably physically ill – went to a workhouse infirmary.

One example is given in the Annual Report about a young girl – perhaps of fourteen or fifteen who is called L.M.L. "This unhappy little waif, like a dog with a bad name, seemed destined for a certain career of crime and calamitous ending. She was committed to Reformatory care for a period of five years. She had confessed to repeated pilfering and acts of destruction, and was given to cutting up her clothing. The record of the family history, however, showed the mother to be of a quiet, easy nature, and the home, one where the children were allowed to do pretty much as they liked. The fact that the child, like the others, looked dirty and neglected, with her hair unbrushed and her toes out of her boots, told their own tale. Homes with vacancies, however, one after another steadily refused the case. At last the Superintendent of the Princess Christian's Farm Colony took pity and consented to give the delinquent a trial. Conditions in which she was understood, resulted in a complete change of demeanour." The Superintendent herself went on to say, "'You ask me about L.M.L., the girl whose case paper was such that it was difficult to find a home for her. On arrival she caused much amusement by her demure ways attached to such a diminutive figure. In a short time she was accepted as the pet child of the Girls' Home, her amusing bouts of mischief being enjoyed by an admiring circle – and the source carefully hidden from authority. The Colony has transformed this black sheep into a ewe lamb."

Families could ask that their relative be accepted and the question of payment was then raised by the Colony's management. There were set fees which parents were expected to pay but there is some indication that, where the parents – or often just the mother – were poor, exceptions were made. However, it is clear that local Councils all over the country could also suggest a person for whom they would pay. The Kent Archives have very little about the Princess Christian Farm Colony and the few documents that they do have relate mainly to 1960-1980. However, there are two minute books of The Kent County Council Mental Deficiency Committee[53] from 1914 to 1930 which cover county-wide issues such as new or expanded mental hospitals. In 1924, for example, a new asylum was proposed at Westwell, near Ashford, at a cost of £201,000. The minutes show that Leybourne Grange Asylum was, by now, with Barming, the main hospital for West & Central Kent and that grants to Princess Christian came via Leybourne. This in turn may indicate that Leybourne was able to send people to Princess Christian – although there is no mention of Princess Christian being a formal subsidiary of Leybourne in any other paperwork until 1949 and the change to the NHS. In 1929, £4,060 was granted by the Committee towards temporary accommodation for ninety-four mentally deficient females and, although it is not mentioned whether the money was for Leybourne or Princess Christian, it must have been for Leybourne because of its large scale.

However, the other main role of the Kent County Council Mental Deficiency Committee was to decide about individuals. Was there a reasonable case for a particular person to be paid for by the Kent County Council in one of the mental homes in the county? There are only two instances in the first one hundred and fifty pages of minutes which relate to the Princess Christian Farm Colony or to Hildenborough. The first concerns Daisy Jackson, aged thirty-three, who in January 1915 is already living at Princess Christian. The Mental Deficiency Committee seems to have been asked to pay for her upkeep. However, the Committee declined on the grounds – and it is not clear exactly what the rules were which led to the decision – that "her mental deficiency did not exist from an early age". Although the only other case does not actually relate to Princess Christian. it does give an indication of how mentally deficient people were treated. In January 1915, Dick Willard is aged nine and lives by coincidence in Hildenborough, at Club Cottages, Riding Lane, just down the road from Princess Christian. He is described as "an imbecile," the medical term of the time indicating a severe type of mental disability. The decision relates to a dispute about how Dick should be helped. The minutes go on to explain.

"The father is opposed to the boy going away to an Institution but the Petition [*presumably a document produced by the local health authorities, probably the Medical Officer for the District*] will be in due course presented to a Judicial Authority for an Order placing him (Willard) into an Institution. The father will have an opportunity of opposing the Order and it will be left to the Judicial Authority to decide the matter." This example of how a 'mad' or 'lunatic' or 'imbecile' person was treated is given because it gives some indication of the care with which the various authorities tried to deal with difficult cases, even if it does not directly relate to the Princess Christian Farm Colony.

Money and the 1920 Fête

In 1920 there appears to have been a financial problem. An article in the Courier of 7 May 1920 reports that Colony was said to be £2,000 in debt – a very large sum – and it had been agreed to hold a two-day fête in June to raise both money and awareness. Dr Frank Fraser, the much respected and well connected doctor from Leigh and the Medical Officer of the Colony – he had been a forceful presence in the neighbourhood for forty years – was made Chairman of the Fête Committee. Princess Christian herself, now a particularly large seventy-five year old and not in particularly good health, was invited to attend and she accepted. The Courier articles from the week leading up to the event give a long list of titled and other VIP guests who were expected to be present. On the day before the opening, Dr Fraser drove around West Kent to pick up journalists in his car – remember how few cars there were in 1920 – for a tour of inspection given by the Superintendent, Miss Pitman, the pivotal figure in the Colony.

In the event, the fête was a little more prosaic, as the Courier reported on 11 June. Princess Christian did not come – it was said she was summoned to Court – but she sent her elder daughter, Princess Marie Louise, who later became the Patron of the Farm Colony. A good number of the titled invitees did not attend either, although the Bishop of Rochester, together with a member of the Astor family, and a good number of more ordinary gentry did. The article is interesting in that it gives another indication of how the 'colonists' spent their time. They provided "plain and fancy articles" for one stall, dairy produce for another, and gave a display of country dancing. The article also shows how the Colony was well supported by the more ordinary residents in the local community. However, there is no mention of how much money was made from this particular fête or how many additional donations were received to help pay off what had been said to be the large bank overdraft.

However, the 1921/22 Annual Accounts for both the National Association and the Farm Colony have been found.[54] Puzzlingly but happily, they show both bodies to be in a healthy financial state. They also provide useful insights into how the Farm Colony was run. The National Association begins the year 1921/22 with £5,000 in hand, with its main outgoings over the year of £800 being for its own administration and salaries – it had to do the overall organization of fourteen homes all over England as well as the Farm Colony. Of the four hundred and forty-five applications received in the year, it had been able to find places for about a quarter. However, it goes on to express concern that more help is not available nationally, particularly for more serious cases, while saying that government money is naturally difficult in the post-war years. Most surprisingly – not least in view of the dire warnings in 1920 – the Annual Report goes on to say that the Association is doing so well that it can reduce the fees it is charging, although the amount of the fees are not given. Accounts for the Farm Colony show a profit over the year of around £1,500 with an income of £7,600, mainly from fees from parents. Expenditure is around £6,000, with £3,500 spent on food/clothing, £1,000 on wages, and £1,400 on rates/maintenance/admin, etc. There are also separate accounts for the Farm itself. Its major earner continued to be milk, butter and eggs (£650), with a smaller amount earned from selling livestock. A footnote adds that £250 of the profit came from providing food grown by the Colony itself – not perhaps a massive contribution in financial terms but useful in providing rewarding work.

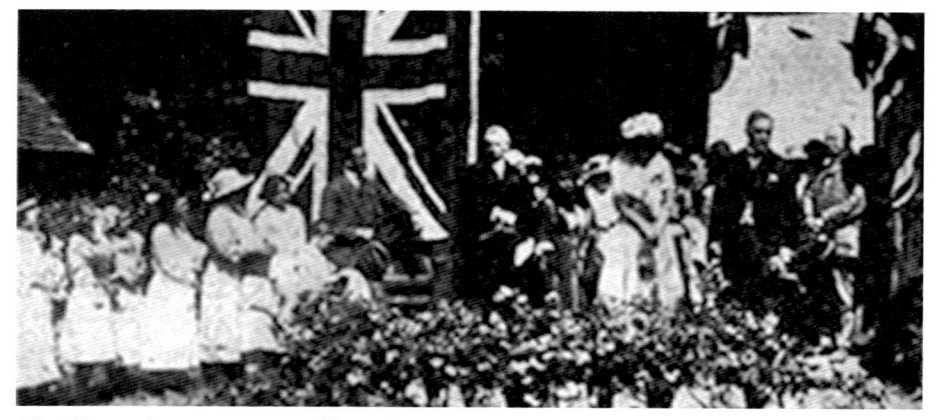

The Fête 11 June 1920 opened by Princess Marie Louise.
Photo: Courier 11 June 1920 by Allwork, Tonbridge.

The Colony always sought to raise money in other ways – firstly from subscriptions and secondly by events. While both must have been useful in raising awareness, neither contributed a huge amount to the overall income. Around two hundred and fifty subscribers are named in the Annual Report but as normally each person gave a guinea, the total contribution was only £300. Similarly, there were summer fêtes each year throughout the 1920s and 1930s. From the various newspaper reports we have of them, on average they seemed to have raised about £30 each. However, they provided a window into the Colony for outsiders. A further source of funds – albeit on a very small scale and usually to help with seaside trips or the Christmas festivities – came from local bodies. The Sevenoaks Guardians of the Poor, established in the 1830s, seemed to give small sums on a regular basis. For example, their Minutes from 10 December 1920 relating to Princess Christian stated, "The usual allowance for the Xmas Extras was allowed." There is also a mention in 1927 of a two shilling grant from the local Sevenoaks Council towards Christmas extras.

A Courier article from 3 August 1928 describes one of the typical events to raise funds. "The Princess Christian Farm Colony presented a festive appearance on Friday when a sale of works was held, the object being to provide the 'colonists' with joys during the holidays, days at the seaside and other pastimes. All goods sold were the works of the 'colonists', who clearly entered the event with considerable enthusiasm under the direction of Miss Pitman, the popular Superintendent. The goods were sold by Miss Banister, the Sewing Mistress, and the 'colonists' themselves. The stalls were arranged in the Pitman Hall and many well-known families in the district were represented. Dr Langdon-Down, Chairman of the Colony, and Mrs Down, motored from Cardiff to attend. The Rev C A Manley was present representing the Vicar, the Rev S G Chamberlen, but the 'colonists' missed an old friend in Dr Frank Fraser, who is away on holiday. The girls gave a well-acted play, entitled 'The Incubus' and in the evening the boys presented 'The King's Escape'. Later the 'colonists' gave an impromptu concert and dancing was also enjoyed. Coconut shies and other amusements were freely patronised. As a result of the sale £29 5s will go to the Joy Fund." Newspaper articles from other years told of the variety of stalls and refreshment tents and about the displays by the 'girls' of folk dancing and of plays they had performed. On one occasion at least there was a drill display by the 'boys'. On another occasion an outside jazz band attended. The fêtes seem to have particularly aimed to raise money to provide funds for special days out. In 1924 the fête raised £28 "in order to pay for the poorer girls' trip to the sea."

Various outside groups were involved with the Colony. The 'boys' played football against the Church Lads Brigade (1925). The Farm entered the Tonbridge Fatstock Show (1914) – a forerunner to the Farm's many entries into agricultural fairs in the 1970s and 1980s. The Tonbridge Amateur Dramatic Society seems to have visited on a fairly regular basis. One newspaper report from just before Christmas in 1929 says the Dramatic Society "presented a successful variety programme which was greatly enjoyed. Two short plays were given, 'The Grand Cham's Diamond' and 'Unbelieving Peter', written by Mr Cyril Cox. Mrs Eric Williams gave a humorous monologue, and later a dialogue with Mrs Budd. Miss Syme rendered violin solos and Miss Catherine French and Mr Cecil Faux songs. Mr Faux acted as accompanist through the evening. The artistes were cordially thanked for their entertainment." What more is there to say!

There are also various mentions in newspapers of St Johns, the Church in Hildenborough and its Vicar, the Rev H J Warde, who was in post from 1918-1924. It seems that there was an informal but a long-term relationship between the Church at the Hildenborough end of Riding Lane and the Colony, a mile and a half up the road, which lasted throughout the Colony's existence until after the Second World War. In the 1921/22 Annual Report Miss Pitman writes, "Thanks are again due to our Vicar, who has been very kind to us throughout the year in arranging Sunday services, both at the Colony and in the Church. More boys and girls have volunteered for the Sunday morning service in the Church, so that to attend has become one of the rewards for good behaviour." It is implied that in addition to these voluntary services in the Church, official Farm Colony services continued to be held on Sunday afternoons in the main hall. When the Rev Warde died in September 1924, there was a mention of his work with the Colony in his obituary. Christmas was also celebrated both with services and with seasonal jollity and a party. The 1921/22 Annual Report says, "Christmas Day falling on a Sunday this year, it was given up to keeping the religious festival, while the other festivities were postponed until the following day." There is also a newspaper report of a Holy Communion service at the Colony just after the start of the Second World War.

So, it is clear that people from the Colony were taken on various trips; that the local community did aim to help; that the kind of folk dancing and plays taught in ordinary schools in the period were taught to the 'colonists'; and that the 'girls' were being taught to sew and make things to sell – seemingly generally being kept well occupied and well cared for.

Dr Reginald Langdon-Down still continued his life-long commitment to Princess Christian with what would have been a longish journey to and from Normansfield.

Death of Jane Langdon-Down in 1917 and Reginald's Remarriage in 1922

Dr Reginald had married Jane Jarvie Cleveland in 1895. Jane at some point – it is not clear exactly when – was in charge of the nursing operation at Normansfield. However, they must have had their first home in Central London – perhaps in Welbeck Street where we know Reginald had his own consulting room at some point (or just possibly at Dr John's original Harley Street consulting rooms) because the birth of their first daughter, Stella, was registered in Marylebone in 1896. That was the year of Dr John's death and, with the increased responsibility at Normansfield, Reginald and his new family seemed to have moved from London to Teddington because the birth of his second daughter, Elspie, in 1899 was registered there. Jane must have had considerable input to the Farm Colony both at the planning stage in the early years of the century and when it became operational in the ten years from around 1907. It must have been a great blow not only to the family but to Normansfield and to the Princess Christian Farm Colony when she died in 1917, leaving her husband and two daughters, but also Jack, their 'mongol' son, without her support.

Five years after Jane's death, Reginald married again.[55] His new wife was Amy Ruth Turnbull – always known as Ruth. She was around forty four years old and, with her sister, Evelyn, had been involved with good works in the Tonbridge area for many years. Ruth had been Commandant of the VAD Hospital in Tonbridge during the Great War and received an MBE for her work in 1920, while Evelyn was in charge of the nursing there. In the early 1920s Ruth had volunteered to organize the 'boys' band at the Colony and must have got to know Reginald well. We know about this from a paragraph by Miss Pitman in the 1921/22 Annual Report. "Owing to the marriage of our kind friend, Miss Turnbull, the 'boys' band is in need of a new leader. Boys and girls were delighted to receive an invitation to her wedding [to Dr Reginald] and all availed themselves to the opportunity to wish her God's blessing…" The variety of other guests at their wedding as reported in the Courier gave an indication of how widely she was involved locally in other ways. We do not know whether she actively participated in the day-to-day running of Princess Christian but, with her experience, it seems likely that at the very least she gave advice over the next twenty years until her death in 1942 and we have one example, given later, where she presided at a ceremony in 1926.

Oversight of the Colony in the 1920s and 1930s

We know something about how the National Association and the Colony were governed in the period immediately after the First World War.56 The previously mentioned National Association's 1921/22 Annual Report lists the seven committees which oversaw the National Association and the Farm Colony. The main Council had thirteen Vice Presidents who included an archbishop, two bishops and many titled ladies and gentlemen. The Medical Committee had fourteen doctors and specialists – including three lady doctors. Amongst the other committees, there was a Colony Sub-Committee which Reginald Langdon-Down chaired; and a Colony Case Sub-Committee over which Sir William Chance presided. The Finance Sub-Committee was overseen by Sir William, with Dr Reginald and three other members. It is clear from the lists of those concerned with the National Association and the Colony that there was a good deal of influence available as well as practical expertise; and the lists in the Annual Report indicate a good balance between general oversight and detailed, specialist knowledge of the feeble-minded. It seems too that, at least in some years, the National Association's meetings were held at the Farm Colony because in 1923 there is a mention that "about a dozen members from London attended the meeting in Hildenborough and were given a tour by Dr Reginald and Miss Pitman."

On the death of Princess Christian in 1923, Princess Marie Louise and her younger sister, Princess Helena Victoria, had taken over patronage of the Farm Colony. There is no record of how much detailed support they gave to either the Farm Colony or to the National Association, although they certainly devoted considerable energy continuing their mother's work to the training of nurses in Britain.

As has been mentioned earlier, there seems to have been a group of three who helped Dr Reginald oversee the Colony sometime in the 1920s and 1930s. The first, and the one who became famous, was Dr Walter Russell Brain, later the 1st Baron Brain. Dr Brain had married Stella, Dr Reginald's elder daughter in 1920 but that was not the only reason he would have been associated with the Colony. He had been to New College, Oxford, studying medicine, qualifying in various specialisms in 1922 and 1923. By 1931 he had been elected as a Fellow of the Royal College of Physicians, of which he became President from 1950-1956. His particular interest was neurology and he served on a number of government committees relating to mental health. (He also looked after Winston Churchill in his final days.) So in the 1920s and 1930s, he was a rising star in the mental health world and would have been able to swap ideas with his father-in-law. The two lady committee members, Dr Reginald's second wife, Ruth and her sister, Miss Evelyn Turnbull, were both 'doers'. As we have seen, they had worked in the Tonbridge VAD Hospital during the Great War. Evelyn, who lived at The Mill House, only a few hundred yards from Princess Christian, became in due course head of VAD units for the whole of Kent. So both sisters had a strong practical and organizing streak which, together with their medical experience, undoubtedly helped the Farm Colony to prosper.

The Death of a Resident 1930

With so few documents to go on, any piece of information helps build up a picture of the Farm Colony. One such article comes from The Courier 31 October 1930. As is so often the case with 'news', it covers an unusual event rather than the everyday life of the Colony. However, the fragility of the residents – whether in 1930 or in 1980 – together with the potential problems faced by staff, are moving. The report of the death of twenty-five year old Thomas Rattenbury is, therefore, given in full.

Courier 31 October 1930

A Midnight Chase
THE SUBSEQUENT TRAGEDY
MENTAL DEFICIENT'S DEATH

The story of a policeman's midnight chase along Tonbridge High-street was described to the Coroner (Mr. Arthur H. Neve) at the inquest held at the Fire Station, Tonbridge, on Wednesday, on Gilbert Thomas Rattenbury, aged 26 years, an inmate of the Princess Christian's Farm Colony, whose body was taken from the Medway early on Wednesday morning.

Thelia Antoinette Koskina, sister-in-charge at Princess Christian's Farm Colony for mental deficients, Hildenborough, said deceased was certified mentally deficient. He had been at the home more than five years.

She saw him at the Colony between 4 and 4.30 on Tuesday. He was of a very low mental order. He had quarrelled with a boy whilst at work during the afternoon and threatened to run away, but the other boy only laughed.

Got Down the Fire Escape

William Stephen Moore, gardener at the Colony, said he had known deceased 5½ years. He thought that the quarrel with the other youth had upset deceased, because the other gardener had told him to stop. Witness was occupying a bedroom near the dormitory to see that everything was all right. Deceased was in bed then. About 11.35 one of the lads knocked at witness's door and said Rattenbury had gone. He found the deceased had gone down the fire escape, and he then searched the premises and finding nothing returned to bed until 5.30, when he had another search. Deceased was a quiet, good tempered lad and on good terms with the rest of the inmates, and had never threatened suicide.

Policeman's Promptitude

PC F.R. Gosling stated that on Tuesday night he was on duty in the High Street, and just before 12.30 he was between the Botany and East-street, when he saw deceased walking in the direction of Tunbridge Wells. Witness called to him "Good Morning" but he did not reply and quickened his pace. Deceased was fully clothed, but had only rubber shoes on. Witness called again to him, but deceased started running very swiftly and witness followed him. Deceased turned in at the River Walk and ran along beside the river with witness following. When about ten yards along witness heard a splash, which sounded about 30 yards away. He was then joined by PC F Smith and both searched the water. About 80 yards from where witness first heard the splash he saw deceased in the water. He procured a shop blind pole, and putting one foot on a stump of wood in the water, with the other policeman holding his hand, managed to reach deceased and pulled him out. Artificial respiration was tried and the doctor and ambulance called. Witness did not think deceased was in the water for more than four minutes. Although artificial respiration was continued, the doctor on arrival announced life extinct. From the inside of the fence on the River Walk to the water were three steps used for rowing boats and it seemed to witness that the deceased thought those steps led into a garden and walked in to the water. The night was very dark and deceased seemed excited.

Dr G. L. Bunting said he was called about 1 a.m. and found the man still warm, but there was no sign of life. There was very little water in his lungs, but he thought death was due to drowning.

The Coroner returned a verdict of "Death by Drowning, there being no evidence to show why or how he came to be in the water." He commended the police on their pluck and promptitude and said that with a bit of luck the deceased's life would undoubtedly have been saved.

Another problem involving the police, although very much less serious, was reported in the local paper six years later in 1936 when two fifteen year old 'boys' from the Colony absconded. They were duly caught "through the initiative of an AA patrol who saw the two boys near Turkey Mill in Maidstone." He reported his suspicions to the police and in due course the boys were caught. However, looked at in the round, in spite of these two cases, there were very few problems with the residents at Princess Christian – or at least very few that were reported in the newspapers.

Medical Treatment 1900-1940

In Victorian times and even until some modest advances in the 1930s and 1950s, medical treatment for people who were thought to be insane or lunatic or feeble-minded was not at all sophisticated. It was reckoned that a disciplined, routine life away from the complexities of society was the best that could be provided. By the 1930s, two treatments had become available for mentally ill people, Electroconvulsive Therapy (ECT), introduced in 1938; and lobotomies, introduced in 1936. Although these types of treatment were used at Leybourne, it does not seem likely that they were needed for the type of patient sent to Princess Christian who predominantly had learning disabilities rather than mental illness. However, in the 1930s and 1940s new drugs were being introduced and these were almost certainly used at Princess Christian. Mild doses of the various barbiturates might have sometimes been used to calm patients down; and amphetamines would probably have been given to help raise some patients' morale – particularly if they were depressed. However, only the more severely ill would have been treated with bromide pills or barbiturates. The normal treatment for the 'colonists' in the 1930s and 1940s continued largely as the founders intended – regimented but essentially kind and well-supervised work on the Farm or in the dairy, in the carpentry workshop or in the gardens, in the laundry, in the kitchens or in the sewing room. The relatively wide range of actual or perceived disabilities continued within the Colony with at least some 'colonists' still put into Princess Christian because of some minor mental or physical difficulty with which their relatives felt they could not cope. However, the problem would continue to be that, after a good number of years in an institution, even such people with little wrong with them originally, would have found it difficult to live in the outside world.

Expansion in the 1920s and 1930s

Expansion at Princess Christian continued. By 1922 the total number of 'colonists' at Princess Christian was one hundred and thirty-nine, with seventy-one boys/men and sixty-eight girls/females. These numbers seem fairly stable, so that in 1926 there were seventy-eight 'boys' and fifty-eight 'girls' and in 1929 there were seventy-one and sixty-three respectively. As well as the conversion of the two cottages into the Hostel in 1922, a more major development occurred between 1924 and 1926. A large new hall was built. What appears to be the original foundation stone of this new building now forms the back of a seat built just outside the main entrance in 2001.

The new hall, although presumably overseen by the National Association's architect, Mr Stewart-Green, was largely erected by the 'colonists' themselves over a two year period. A newspaper article[57] gives a good idea of the eventual building which was named the Pitman Hall in honour of Miss Pitman, the Superintendent or Principal of the Colony for so many years. "The Hall was about 75 yards from the main building. It is built in bungalow style of red brick, with red tiled roof. Entrance can be made by two doors and two French windows, while the hall itself is well supplied by windows. The hall is 90ft by 40ft and the woodwork and the floor is of pitch pine. At one end of the hall is an altar, complete with flowers and fittings, which can be closed up when not in use. Over the altar is a painting of the Madonna and the Holy Babe. At the other end of the room is a good-sized stage and dressing rooms are also provided ... On the right hand wall hang two oil paintings, one of Sir William Chance, Chairman of the National Association, and the other of Dr Frank Fraser of Leigh, the Medical Attendant of the Institution. Both are taken from photographs, and painted by one of the boys." The formal opening of the Pitman Hall at the end of June 1926 was clearly a grand event. The Bishop of Rochester, ever a friend of the Farm Colony, and his chaplain, together with the Rural Dean and a number of local clergy, all in their robes and followed by the local gentry, together with the staff and residents at the Colony, all walked in a procession from the main building to the Hall. The Bishop, in dedicating the Hall and its altar, praised the management of the Colony and wished the whole enterprise well. All the visitors were then taken on a tour of the Colony. There was further building work in the first part of the 1930s but we have no details. In 1935 it was the Colony's Jubilee Year – twenty-five years since 1910 – when there were apparently considerable celebrations, although again we have no details.

From the Start of an Idea to The Second World War

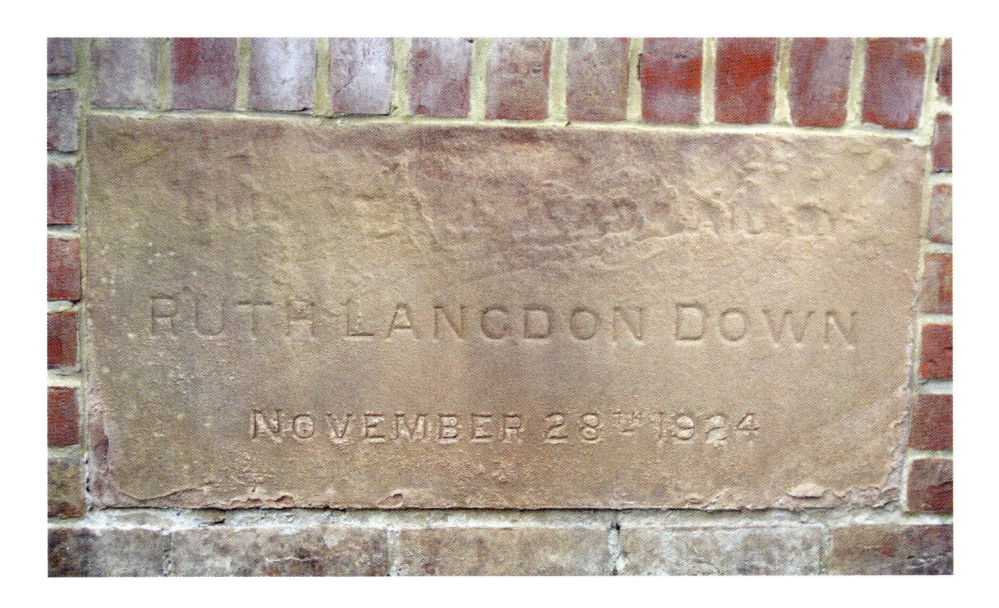

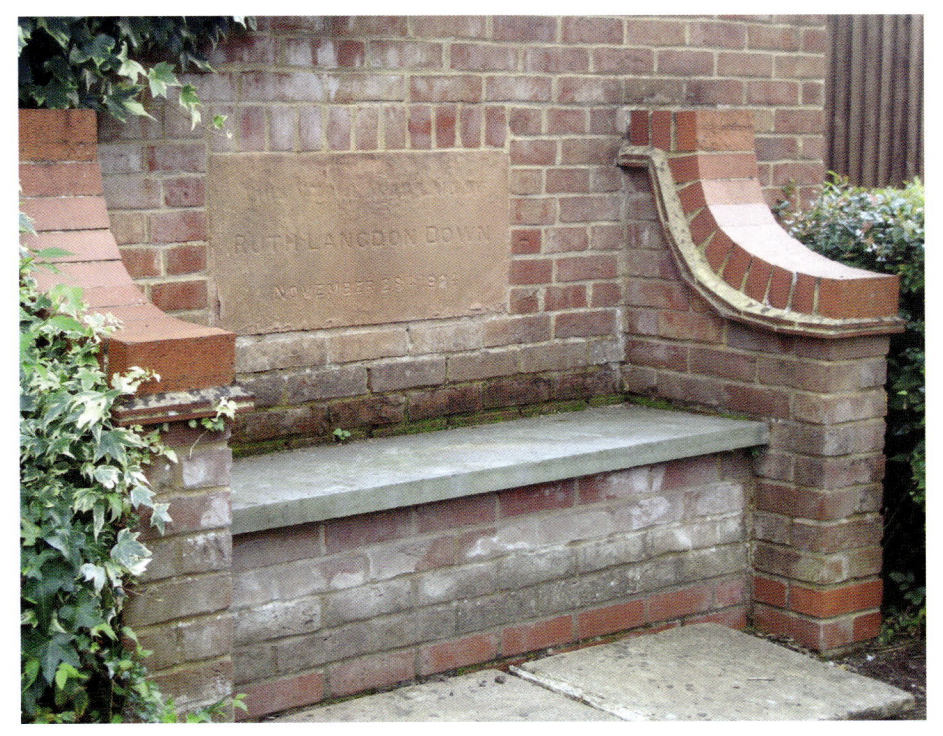

Above: Apparent foundation stone of a building opened on 28 November 1924 by Ruth Langdon-Down, Dr Reginald's second wife.
Photos: Anna Rowley

At some stage in the early 1930s Dr Reginald Langdon-Down seems to have decided to sell Oaklands. He probably thought that he did not use the house often enough to justify the expense. In any case, the house was put up for sale. Soon after, the estate agent reported back that there was little interest in country houses currently and that he could find no buyers.

By 1932 some newspaper articles show that the house was rented out as an "International Centre". Presumably the Centre did not flourish, because a year or two later "the premises were opened to hikers, providing lodging accommodation at very low charge." At this stage the National Association decided that it wanted to buy the house. They wanted to convert it for some extra 'girls' whom they wanted to move from an Association home in Uxbridge called Alexander House which was being closed. The problem was that the Association seems to have assumed that it could make the change without much consultation. When the plans became more public, the neighbours complained. The issue went before the Tonbridge Town Planning Joint Committee on 2 April 1937 presided over by the rather splendidly named Major C G Field Marsham. The Association seems to have put forward this application without mentioning that the house was to be part of the Princess Christian Farm Colony and without approaching any of the neighbours in what was – and still is – a relatively upper class road and area. What was called "a home for backward girls" was not likely to be instantly popular. Consequently, the Council wrote to the owners of the four nearest houses to ask their views. All opposed the proposal and Major Field Marsham said "he personally thought it would be rather a hardship on the owners." The application was therefore refused. The National Association appealed this decision. This time, their case was better prepared. The appeal was held at Tonbridge Castle and an outsider, Mr H R Wardill, an inspector at the Ministry of Health, conducted the inquiry. The National Association had brought in its own lawyer and called witnesses including Dr Reginald Langdon-Down. The newspaper reported that Dr Reginald clarified the original proposal and explained that "while the female defectives at the main Princess Christian Farm Colony were certified under the Mental Deficiency Act, it was proposed to receive at Oaklands only high-grade, uncertified defective girls and women." He went on to emphasize that, as far as he knew, over many years the managers at the Farm Colony had never received any complaints from neighbours. The National Association's lawyer went on to claim that property prices had not been affected by the main Princess Christian buildings and the use of Oaklands by the Princess Christian Farm Colony would similarly not affect the value of local houses. The Tonbridge Rural Council's lawyer strongly disputed the claims. "The proposed use was likely to be repugnant to the residential users of the area and detrimental to local interests." He called a good number of witnesses including an estate agent who claimed property values *would* be affected. However, after all this very British and very lengthy consultation process, permission was finally given (perhaps it helped having an inspector who was from the Ministry of Health) and the National Association was able to buy Oaklands which it re-named Alexander House after the home in Uxbridge where the new inmates had previously lived. There is some indication that most of the villagers in Hildenborough were not upset by the decision. The Colony with which they seemed to be at ease was just up the road and they were prepared to help. For example, in the Minute Book of the Hildenborough Men's Club for 1925/26 there is a proposal to donate some of the Club's library books. (In the event, the offer was not taken up by the Colony but it showed a readiness by the ordinary villagers to support Princess Christian).[58] Dr Reginald finally sold Oaklands, which he had owned for twenty-five years but had certainly not used it since at least 1931/32. He continued to remain at his main home near Normansfield but his concern for the Princess Christian Farm Colony never faltered. He died aged eighty-eight in 1955. However, the family involvement continued. His son, Antony, who really did live in Hildenborough, succeeded him as Chairman of the Colony and was – like his father – totally committed for many years to the Princess Christian ideal.

1939-1948

We do not have any formal record of what happened during the war years but the number of 'boys' and 'girls' was somewhat reduced, not least because Alexander House was taken over by the Army. (The Army did a good deal of damage and Alexander House did not re-open until 1952.) We know that at the start of the War, the residents were all fitted with gas masks and Princess Christian staff were trained to be air-raid wardens.[59] However, the work of the Colony and the Farm went on and there were occasional advertisements in the newspapers for staff. It was probably not easy to find the required stockman in January 1940, with the younger men being called up for the Forces and when every farmer was short of trained staff and already relying on inexperienced Land Army girls.

After the War, there were more advertisements in the local papers for staff, but on a larger scale as the organization was able to expand again. For example, on 6 August 1948, an advertisement appeared in the Courier for seven jobs. It seems that the National Health Service had not yet taken over Princess Christian and that the new jobs came under the original charity. The wording gives a picture of the Colony in the immediate post-War era.

The following staff are urgently required:-

- *1 Laundress   £4 per week*
- *1 Domestic Assistant   £3-14s per week*
- *1 Maintenance Man able to drive car and do general running repairs to the Colony   £4-16s per week (Res).*
  [The word 'Res' presumably meant that the man could have accommodation].

These appointments subject to Superannuation where applicable.
A deduction of £1-3s per week is made for board and lodging if resident.

- *1 Farm Labourer   £5 per week*
- *1 Gardener   £4-16s per week*
  Subject to Superannuation
  Medical Examination

- *1 Male Nurse*
- *I Female Assistant Nurse*
  Salary according to Rushcliffe scale according to experience
  Full residential emoluments
  Subject to Superannuation
  Medical Examination

Applications to the Lady Superintendent of the Colony

This advertisement appears by permission of the Ministry of Labour and National Service under the Control of Engagement Order 1947.

So, it is clear from this last sentence that at a time when labour was extremely short, the authorities considered Princess Christian worthwhile and it was allowed to advertise for new staff. The 'Lady Superintendent' must have been the long-serving and redoubtable Miss Pitman and this would have been one of her last tasks at Princess Christian. As we will see, a new superintendent was brought in when the National Health Service eventually took over.

The Views of Local Residents 1900-1949

The local community had accepted the Farm Colony which had grown from a small start in 1907/08 to a relatively large part of the Hildenborough scene forty-five years later. It is not known how many local people the Colony employed to look after and teach its approximately one hundred and forty 'colonists' between the Wars but it must have been one of the district's major employers with maybe up to forty or fifty full-time and part-time staff.

The reports about objections at the Oaklands' Planning Inquiry might seem to indicate that local people were antagonistic to the Colony. However, this does not seem to have been the case. Even the neighbours who opposed the new use for Oaklands said that there had never been cause for complaint and seemed hesitant to further criticize the Colony itself. This feeling that the Colony was part of the fabric of the area is echoed by locals who can remember back to the 1930s and 1940s. The pre-war regime was described by one local man, Bob Duffin, who grew up in The Club Cottages, half a mile down Riding Lane from the Farm during the late 1920s and the 1930s. "Miss Pitman was still the Superintendent all through the 1930s. She was a sort of Margaret Rutherford type from the 'Doctor in the House' films, very strict and very much in charge. Parents were allowed to visit once a year – not at all like it was in the 1960s onwards when the new type of people in charge encouraged the parents and the local community to come to see what was happening and aimed to get them involved. But the staff were really caring – or nearly always. Bill Hobden was the Farm Manager before the War – the Farm was almost opposite us. He was a typical member of the staff at Princess Christian. Good at looking after and training the 'colonists' but good at the farming side too. He lived at Brownway Cottage in Riding Lane, and during the War he married Moira who was a Land Girl locally. I used to see the 'boys' and 'girls' almost every day. They were in their crocodiles – separate for 'boys' and 'girls' – walking down Riding Lane with their own nurse attendant. And, as my school days at Hildenborough Primary progressed, I got to know quite a few of them and they'd call out 'Morning Bob'; 'Hello Bob'. In spite of the sense of regimentation, I still think that the 'boys' and 'girls' enjoyed their lives there." And Bob adds another memory which may illustrate how closely the local community and the Farm Colony were involved with each other, even before the Second World War. In the later 1930s, when Bob was a teenager, he became interested in the cinema. He wanted to show some of his school friends a film he had obtained. Even though he lived half a mile down Riding Lane, he thought it perfectly easy to go to the Farm Colony authorities whom he knew quite well and ask if he could use one of the brick buildings just inside the gates of Alexander House as a cinema. They agreed without any concern. (And although the film only lasted a minute or two, Bob charged his friends an entrance fee!)

So the Farm and the main Colony were an ordinary part of life in the Hildenborough area, and to this day the 'colonists' of the 1930s, 1940s and 1950s are remembered with affection.

The Lack of Records about the Princess Christian Farm Colony

For the first thirty or forty years of the Farm Colony there are almost no records about the staff or the patients or how it was run, apart from the initial 1911 census details and the 1921/22 National Association's Annual Report and Accounts. It may well be that all the paperwork for the 1904 to 1948 period was passed over to the NHS when The Colony became 'The Hospital' around 1949 or 1950. However, one local resident who worked at Princess Christian for over twenty years in the NHS period has said that it was a standing joke amongst staff that the NHS threw away the pre-1949 records. And added – and we will never know to what extent it happened – that most or many NHS records were also disposed of as Princess Christian was wound down between 1990 and 1993 and the organization for the former 'colonists' principally passed from the NHS to Kent County Council Social Services. The suspicion that the NHS did not pass on any records was supported by a senior social worker. In 1995, he asked the NHS about a seventy-five year old man who had come from Leybourne Grange to Princess Christian. His records from the NHS days were kept, he was told, by the KCC Social Services. In any case, as all NHS records are confidential, it is perhaps not surprising that no medical or organizational records have been available from the NHS. So, this first part of the book, from around 1900 to around 1949, has had to rely heavily on the views of people who knew the Colony – luckily informative and often moving – together with isolated newspaper reports. However, the next part of this book, which covers the NHS years, contains not only first-hand memories but a few official documents which describe life at the Princess Christian Hospital from 1949/50 onwards.

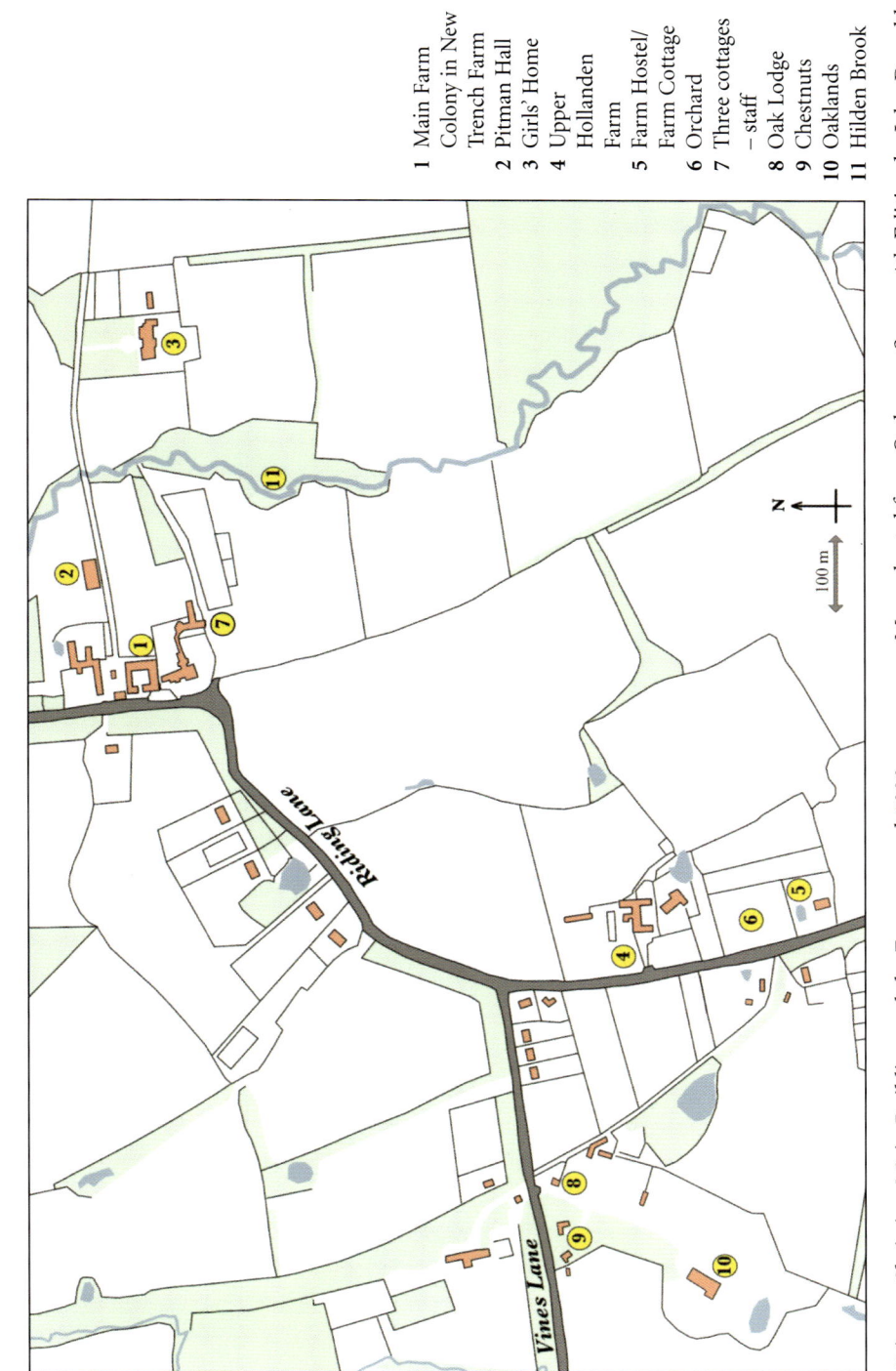

1 Main Farm Colony in New Trench Farm
2 Pitman Hall
3 Girls' Home
4 Upper Hollanden Farm
5 Farm Hostel/Farm Cottage
6 Orchard
7 Three cottages – staff
8 Oak Lodge
9 Chestnuts
10 Oaklands
11 Hilden Brook

Princess Christian Main Building and the Farm around 1938.   *Map adapted from Ordnance Survey 4th Edition by John Donald*

CHAPTER 3

From the Second World War until the early 1980s

The National Health Service Takes Over

The National Health Service formally started on 5 July 1948 but it seems it was sometime in 1949 or even 1950 that the NHS took over the Princess Christian Hospital – as it then became known. During and immediately after the Second World War, the Farm Colony had been run much as it had been for the previous forty years. The 'boys' and 'girls' were now formally known as 'patients'. Quite a number had what later became called Down's syndrome. Others had various degrees of autism or epilepsy or deformity or had just been considered inconvenient at some point over the previous forty years. The 'boys' mainly continued to work on the farm. The 'girls' worked in the laundry or at sewing or other domestic work when they were capable of doing so. However, the average age of both 'boys' and 'girls' would have become older with increasing numbers less able to work. By 1950, those who had first come to the Farm Colony in 1910 to 1920 as genuine boys and girls would have been around sixty, if they had survived. What were by now called 'mentally retarded' often died relatively young, even until the 1950s and 1960s. Until this time, the organization had continued to be funded by donations and what the Colony could earn. Some of the more able 'boys' and 'girls' sometimes helped with work in local homes and gardens. A few had left to work in the outside world – often on farms: but not many.

After the move to the NHS, a new Superintendent was appointed. It seems likely to have been a Mr Russell because he was definitely in the post in 1952, according to one article.[60] New patients were increasingly chosen by the Leybourne Grange Hospital doctors and were meant to be classified as 'Category E' patients. This meant that they were "safe and able to be trained." (It was only in 1964 that the connection with Leybourne was formalized and all new patients at Princess Christian came via Leybourne.) New forms of treatment were gradually introduced and some modernization was undertaken, although it was only in the early 1950s that electric irons were installed for the 'girls' to do the ironing and proper sinks introduced into the Girls' Home kitchens for the laundry. Modernization certainly did not come quickly.

Leybourne Grange Hospital 1960-1980

With the paucity of official papers about the treatments and organization of Princess Christian, it is worth using some of the few documents that have recently been found which relate to Leybourne, particularly relating to the early 1970s.[61] In 1973 Leybourne described itself as "a hospital for the mentally subnormal – or to use an older phrase, the mentally deficient." It is clear that forty years ago, no one was quite sure what to call their patients – something which was true a hundred years earlier and still concerns people today. Leybourne's own description of itself goes on to say that "many of these unfortunate people who are mentally subnormal have other handicaps as well, such as physical deformities, behaviour disorders or epilepsy… [They are] of both sexes and of all ages from infancy onwards.

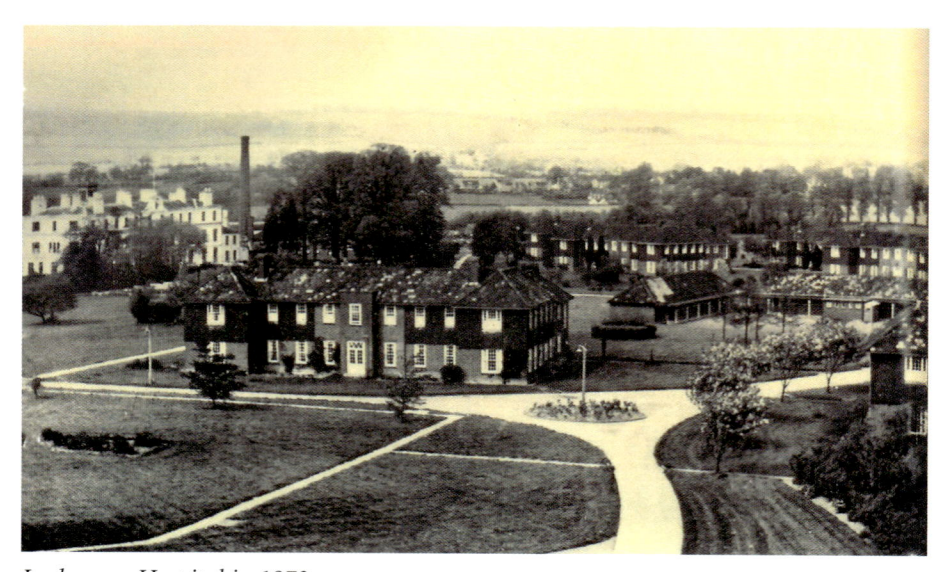

Leybourne Hospital in 1973

From The Second World War Until The Early 1980s

They are also of all degrees of mental sub-normality, from those who can do nothing whatever for themselves up to those whom we can train to be practically independent and to do simple sheltered jobs, by which they may eventually be able to support themselves out in the community." It was this last category of adults which Leybourne would choose – after assessment – to come to Princess Christian.

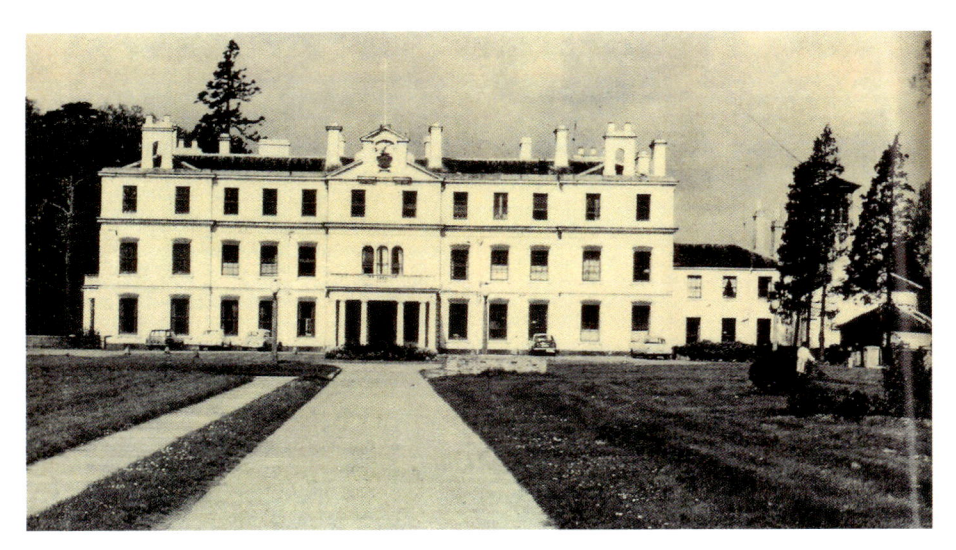

Leybourne Hospital in 1973

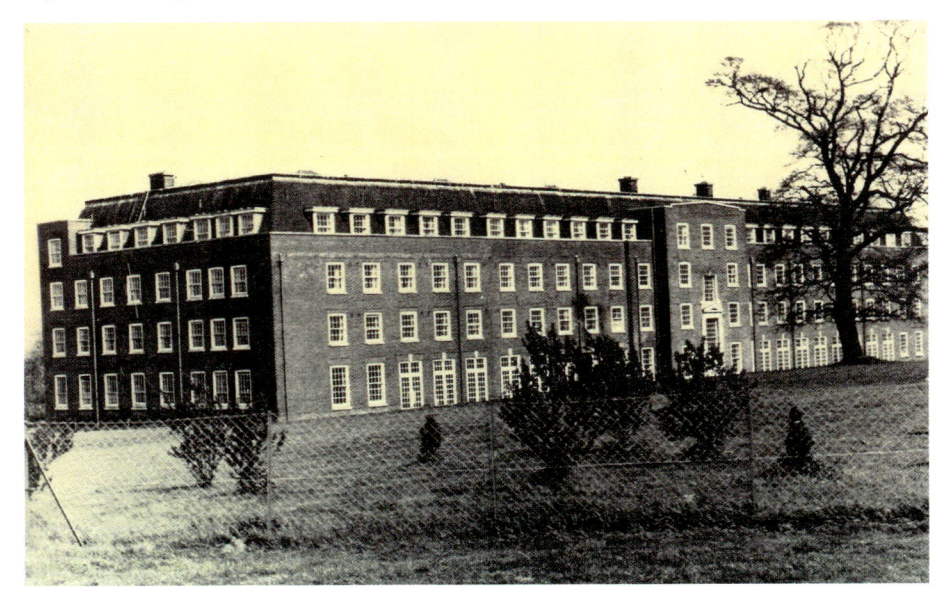

Looking at the wider national picture, it seems that the problems of mental health were grave at the time – the 1960s and 1970s. Leybourne Grange was typical. It could not really cope with the existing numbers satisfactorily, yet it had a long waiting list. It was felt by all concerned with learning disabilities that this type of adversity had in the words of the Lord Aberdare, Ted Heath's Minister of Health and Social Security[62] "suffered for too many years from a lack of public interest as well as resources." He, of course – as with every politician ever since – promised his Party would improve matters. He went on to give a lucid summary of what would be needed, including developing the relatively new policy of 'Care in the Community'. However, he did add, "It will probably take fifteen to twenty years before we have the service that we need." This assessment of the timescale made in June 1973 was perceptive. It was, indeed, between 1988-1993 when Princess Christian and Leybourne were being wound down.

In spite of a number of similarities, Leybourne in 1973 was very different from Princess Christian in a number of ways – particularly its size and the severity of a good proportion of its residents' disabilities. Leybourne was eight or nine times the size of Princess Christian. As one article[63] noted, "It has 1,100 patients or 'residents' as we prefer to call them." The article went on to give more details. There were ten Nursing Officers, 66 Ward Sisters, 90 State Registered Nurses, with a total of 545 nursing staff and 95 trainees. The extent of its buildings – based on the old Leybourne Grange Manor House with its 260 acres – can be seen in the photographs below. The description adds, in order to emphasize the size of the Leybourne organization, that it "has a catering budget of £137,000" (although it does not say whether this was for a week, a month or a year).

The contrast between the two organizations was not just in size. The specialists that were needed at Leybourne for the residents with their varied ages and a wide range of physical and mental disabilities were on a completely different scale to Princess Christian. For example, Leybourne had a school to cope with the children, "often who have been at the hospital since birth and often with inherited disorders." Mrs Louvine Brooks had been the school's headmistress for twenty-three years in 1973 and had a staff of twelve. There was also education for adults. As will be apparent when looking at Princess Christian's educational provision, Leybourne was massively more structured. The children at the Leybourne school would, where possible, be trained so that they could go into the Leybourne workshops when they were about sixteen. Then at around nineteen they would be reassessed to see if they could go out into the community, always the Hospital's aim. Although no confirmation was given in the article, it was probably in this second assessment that the option of sending them to Princess Christian was considered. However, it was assumed that a large proportion of 'the residents' would be at Leybourne for the rest of their lives, looked after by its specialist staff of nurses, therapists and doctors, sometimes with individual nurses caring for individual residents for twenty or thirty years.

The specialist services at Leybourne, whether to help psychological or physical problems (often a combination of both), were also much more professional and varied than at Princess Christian. So, for example, the physiotherapy and occupational therapy departments at Leybourne were large in order to deal with the wide variety of mental and physical disabilities of the residents as well as the sheer numbers. People who were chosen to go to Princess Christian were all more or less physically able-bodied when they arrived. Similarly, the psychology department at Leybourne was very different from anything at Princess Christian. From 1970 on, this department was run by an American psychologist, who had come to England because he had objected to the Vietnam War. He was dubious of the advantages of a large organization like Leybourne. "We are very conscious that work inside the Hospital is made difficult by the Institution itself. Psychologists have to try to minimize the damage that the Hospital does to them. Our future is outside Leybourne and all the other hospitals like them." However, this perhaps simplistic view was echoed, although from an entirely different view point by a new arrival who came as a junior member of the Leybourne staff. Nina Connor was the daughter of the Senior Staff Registered Nurse at Princess Christian, Nan Connor. We will hear more of Nan Connor's story later but her daughter, Nina, has strong views about Leybourne Grange in the 1970s and it is, therefore, sensible to add them at this point. Not surprisingly, having been brought up at Princess Christian, Nina had first become a nursing assistant there, before moving to Leybourne to train as a Staff Nurse.

"When I got to Leybourne in 1978, I felt as though I had stepped back into the Victorian era. The place was clean but the way the patients were cared for was very much the same as the routine that the Victorians had started a hundred years ago. The patients slept in dormitories, up to ten in each one, with very little space between the beds. The only space they had for possessions was a locker and these would be tidied by domestic staff while the patients were out at their daytime activities, giving the patients no part in organizing their own private space and lives. All activities were regimented, with early rising times and set bedtimes regardless of individual needs. Staff would 'shepherd' patients into the bathroom by calling them from the breakfast table. At any one time there could have been up to five or six people in different stages of their ablutions with one staff member to undress, another wash and one to dry them. Privacy and dignity were not recognized as a right or a need – such concepts were not even considered in the 1970s and early 1980s. Staff would walk into the bathroom without knocking or identifying themselves in advance to speak to a staff member on a routine matter or even to have a social conversation. Lack of respect was the norm. Their routine was 'set in stone' to such an extent that people with moderate and severe learning disabilities with challenging behaviour were totally conditioned to their routines, knowing exactly what to do and where to go at any stage of their day. My thoughts around this point in my training were that patients were all treated in an immature and disrespectful manner. The use of language was childlike, with toys and teddies being encouraged. There was no time for people to be recognized as individuals or requiring privacy. They were not expected to have any self-determination or to exercise choice and they were definitely shown very little respect. During my years at the hospital I can recall several incidents of obvious abuse taking place. Pubic hair of women patients was pulled as a way of getting them to comply; and I also saw several patients hit with wet towels. And there were occasions when food was withheld. This unacceptable behaviour appeared to be condoned by the system and was seen to be normal at the time. Inexperience and my junior rank left me in an untenable position and I felt completely unable to change these patterns of work This was the point at which I realized that in the future my aim would be to try and improve the care and well-being of patients."[64] However, Nina did add to her recollections of Leybourne. "It is important to note that not all aspects of this Institution were bad. Some staff took more interest than others with the patients, giving them more time and care. There were also all manner of activities available. Most nights of the week, there were clubs to go to and films, discos, quizzes, etc. All the activities were enjoyed and well attended by the patients." Ten years later Nina Connor, by that time Mrs Nina Brannan, returned to Princess Christian and her account of that time is given later.

Yet another view of Leybourne was taken by one of Leybourne's top medical experts, consultant Dr John Corbett. He completely accepted the coming of 'Care in the Community' and, in the longer term, the proposed closure of Leybourne, with its patients being encouraged to live life as normally as possible in the outside world. However, he had doubts about how fast and how far the process should go. "There is a danger that many small units scattered throughout the community may become equally institutionalized, although in a different way. The need is to set up smaller units varying between 20 and 100 places, where the local community can be more intimately involved in the future well-being of their own mentally handicapped people and staff can be more easily recruited ... [There would also need to be some units acting] as sheltered communities for the older patients... and some highly specialised facilities for the treatment and research into more difficult and complex handicaps."[65] The main document about Leybourne does not give details of the variety of specialists that were available there and were theoretically also available to look after the residents at Princess Christian. However, from other papers, the involvement of Leybourne specialists at Princess Christian does not appear to have been thought necessary very often, possibly because the Leybourne experts chose those who were to go to Princess Christian *because* they were not suffering from the most difficult symptoms or from particular physical problems.

Because this special June 1973 Kent Messenger supplement about Leybourne was aimed at the general public and wanted to involve the public as much as possible with the Hospital, a good deal of information is given about how ordinary people did already and could in the future help with the patients. There were dedicated full-time staff to organize the volunteers from the community, which included regular visits from schools in Sevenoaks, Tonbridge and Maidstone. Leybourne was clearly not only very keen to involve the local community but wanted to try to show how most of the patients were ordinary, non-frightening people. As we shall see, this conscious policy of demystifying the Institution and showing local people that the patients were all individuals, with often gentle characters of their own, was echoed at Princess Christian – partly one suspects because the mother hospital, Leybourne, was infused with the idea, but partly because the principle was 'in the air' nationally as a common-sense progression about mentally retarded people. However, as we will also see, change did not come easily or quickly.

The Mental Health Act 1959

In the 1950s and into the 1960s, the national system was that most patients receiving care for mental illness or mental incapacity had to be assessed formally to establish whether they were receiving the appropriate care for their condition and whether they should be in a hospital or not. However, the whole system was out-dated and underfunded. A series of exposés by the media led to the 1959 Mental Health Act which imposed various reforms on mental institutions and homes for what were now called the 'subnormal', including much more formalized assessments for individual patients. Nationally, quite a number of patients were identified as not needing to be in full hospital care. In the case of Princess Christian Hospital, it was found that several patients should not be in hospital and a few were discharged into the community, supervised and helped by the KCC's Social Services until they had adapted to living away from the hospital environment. Where possible, they were given help into employment. There were also patients who did not need to be in hospital but who had clearly become institutionalized after many years at the Colony, or, as it was now, the Hospital. They continued to live at Princess Christian, as it was considered that it would be cruel and traumatic for them to be uprooted from their long-established home.

One story illustrates how haphazard the choices of who ended up at Princess Christian could be.[66] Derek Bance was born in South London in October 1936. He was illegitimate and was removed from his mother and put into care. One suspects that he was a bit 'slow' – what we would today classify as very mildly autistic – and so was moved to a disabled home where he stayed – institutionalized – until his late teens. He was then transferred to Princess Christian in the 1950s. It must have been clear to the Princess Christian staff that Derek was not as 'mentally retarded' (in the wording of the time) as most of the other 'boys' and he was given a room of his own in the Oast House above the medical centre. At this point, Robin Ballard takes up the story. Robin was the teenage son of Bob Ballard, the engineer at the Hospital from 1947 until 1961. Robin used to go to talk with Derek, not least because Derek had started collecting pop records (78 rpm) which they both loved. Robin got to know Derek well and describes him as being a lovely man with a great sense of humour. Derek had considerable freedom to do what he wanted. He was allowed to go down to Hildenborough each day to collect the newspapers. He often went to the Tonbridge Market where he was well known. But his lifelong passion was for cricket and for many years he was the scorer at the Hildenborough Cricket Club. Eventually, the authorities decided that Derek could cope with life away from the Princess Christian Hospital and he was one of the earlier 'boys' to be moved into his own home, a house with three others in St Mary's Road, Tonbridge organized by KCC Social Services. The story did have a happy ending but Derek Bance's early experience provides an indication not only of the variety of people at Princess Christian but also of how some people, with not very much 'wrong' with them, could end up there, quite often because there seemed no alternative.

The Colony Recovers After the War

Robin Ballard also provides a fuller picture of the Princess Christian Farm Colony in the years just after the War. His father, Bob, had always been interested in mechanical things and, after serving in the RAF during the War, he went to work at the Rawsons car dealership and garage in Tonbridge before getting the job at the Hospital. Initially, he lived in rooms at the main hospital building but in June 1949, when he got married, he and his wife moved to a Princess Christian house, Stone Lodge in Vines Lane. Their son, Robin, was born there in 1951 and their daughter, Paula, in 1956. Both went to the Hildenborough Church of England Primary School.

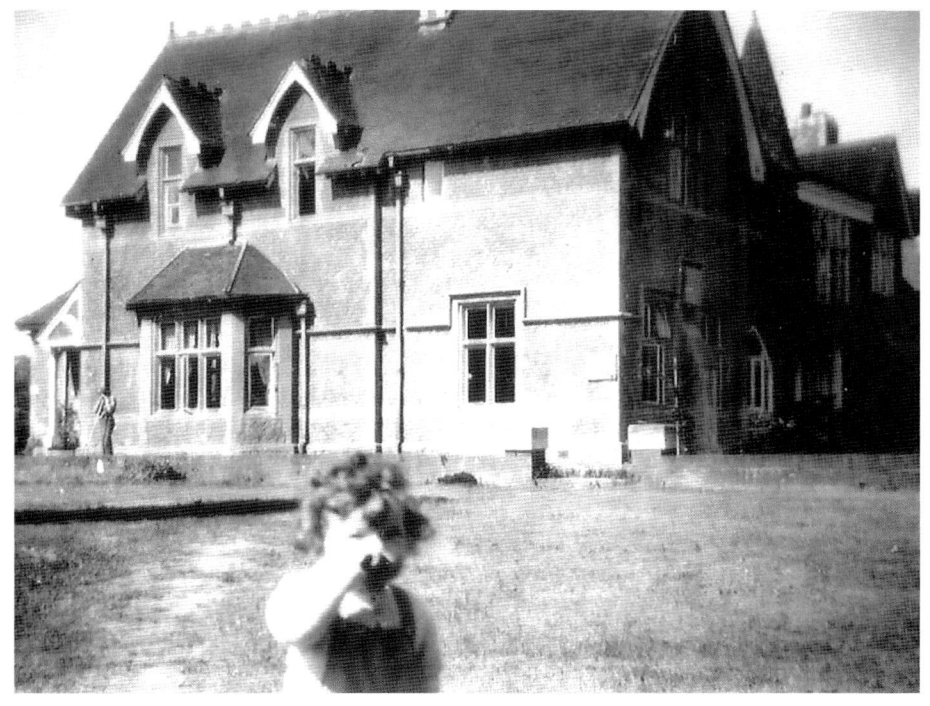

Robin Ballard, aged about 2, around 1953, at the south-west end of Alexander House

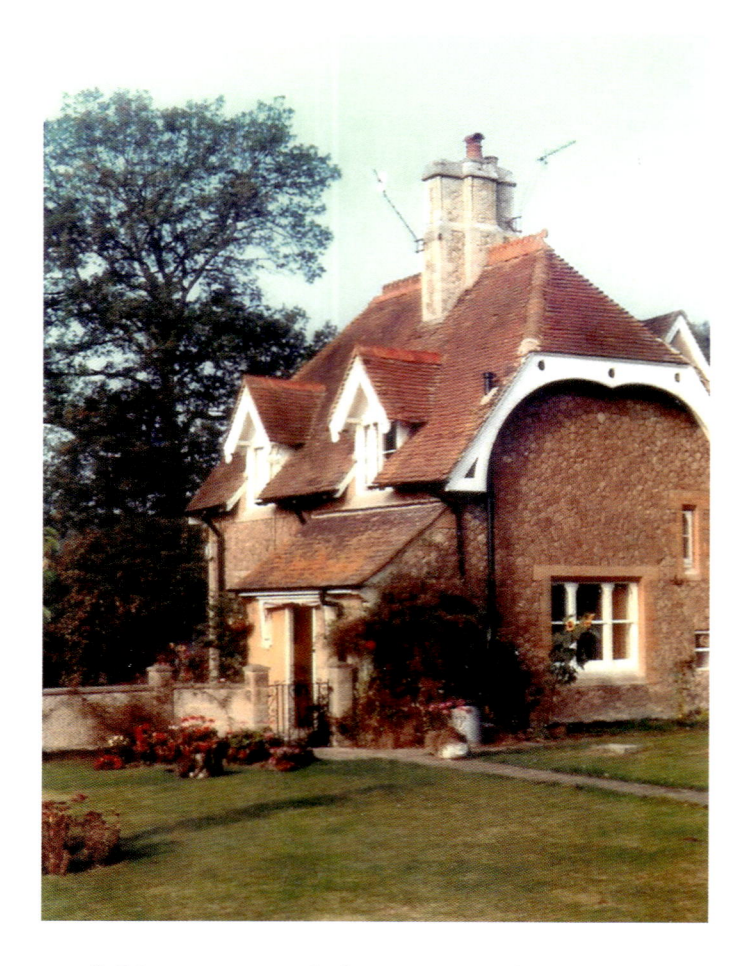

The Princess Christian Farm Colony and Hospital 1895–1995

Stone Lodge in Vines Lane – home of Robin Ballard and his family

"Things were tough for everyone after the War, including the Hospital," says Robin. "Rationing continued until about 1954. The Hospital did not have central heating and it was very difficult to keep the many buildings warm. And most of the buildings needed considerable modernization. But over the years my father introduced an ongoing programme of improvements. The Hospital had its own painter, bricklayer, carpenter, stoker and one engineering assistant, although outside contractors were used for the larger upgrades. New boilers for central heating were installed around the early 1960s. The first replacement ones used solid fuel, burning anthracite grains and they had to be stoked twice a day. The clinker had to be cleared out of the boiler each morning using very long pokers to break the clinker into manageable pieces. Then long handled tongs were used to lift the red hot clinker out of the boiler into large metal coal scuttles which were

From The Second World War Until The Early 1980s

placed outside to cool. The fuel hoppers had to be filled in the morning but also in the late afternoon so that there was sufficient fuel for the boilers to operate until the following day. The boilers were eventually converted to gas in the 1970s. Then there were isolated incidents which involved extra work. There was a serious fire at Alexander House in about 1961. It caused considerable damage to the roof and the two gables to the front of the building. The blaze could be seen from Mill Lane and it lit up the sky. Fortunately, the fire occurred in the evening when the residents were at the Pitman Hall watching a film and there were no casualties. The residents from Alexander House had to spend the night in the Pitman Hall and then alternative accommodation was arranged while the damage was repaired which took several months to complete.

One member of staff from the 1950s whom I particularly remember was Harold Neasham, who was dedicated to looking after the 'boys' at Alexander House. During the summer, he would often play cricket with them on fine evenings. Around 1958 he bought a 1940s Packard limousine from Lord Hollenden in Leigh. It was finished in dark blue paintwork with luxurious upholstery and, although I think the car must have been brought over from the USA, it was right hand drive. It had a glass privacy screen behind the front seats. One Christmas he drove us to London to see the lights in Regent Street and Oxford Street, a real treat in those days. He left Princess Christian in the early 1960s to become a probation officer in one of the London boroughs but for several years he would visit the patients at Alexander House during the evenings. He would call on us first at Stone Lodge and leave his car for me to wash and earn some pocket money. But by then, he was driving such cars as a Hillman Minx and a Singer Gazelle."

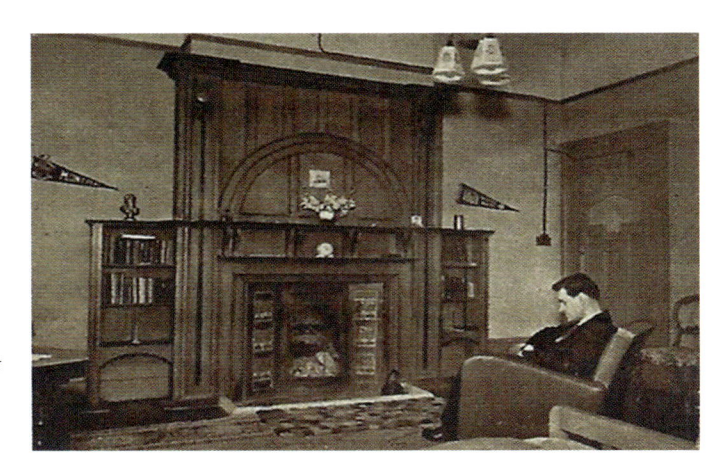

Staff sitting room at Alexander House.
From Nursing Mirror, May 1952.

The Princess Christian Colony and Its Farm in the 1950s

The Farm at Princess Christian might at first sight seem an unusual feature for a mental hospital. Neither Normansfield nor Leybourne had an equivalent. An important principle of the Colony from the start had been to give useful employment to those with mental difficulties. However, the idea was not new. Many Victorian workhouses had not only a farm but a bakery, a cobbler, a laundry and workshops so that inmates, particularly the young, could be trained to live a useful life in the outside world; and some of the large Victorian lunatic asylums had similar facilities where the more able worked or were taught to work, even if they were unlikely to be allowed to be released. Throughout the life of Princess Christian, the Farm was a central feature, mainly for the men, although a few of the women also worked there. It was very important that the Farm was well run. It did not matter whether the Farm was organized by the original charity or by the NHS, or later by the Kent Social Services: there had to be experienced farm managers who could constructively help the residents work with the animals – which they loved – or in the fields, gardens or greenhouses. With few official documents about Princess Christian available, it is lucky that there are a number of individuals who have memories of how the newly-named 'Hospital' and its Farm worked on a day-to-day basis. Robin Ballard, growing up at the Colony, remembers a great deal about the people who worked there. Other particularly interesting first hand sources have been Senior Nurse, Nan Connor, and her daughter Nina, who years later also became a senior manager there; and Joy Dolling (née Burgess) who knew the Mason family well.[67] Mr Edward Mason, always known as 'Ted', became, as we will see, the Superintendent at the Colony. Much information in the following section comes from these four people and the author is most grateful for their help. There is also a Nursing Mirror article from 1952.

The Nursing Mirror article about the Princess Christian Colony on 16 May 1952 contained details of the Farm as well as the overall organization.[68] At the Farm, there was a TT attested herd of cows with over fifty pedigree Ayrshire cattle. There were also some pigs, a lot of chickens and some geese.

Joy Dolling was aged about eight in the early 1950s. She remembers going to the milking parlour to watch the relatively new milking machines in operation. "Most of the milk was consumed by the patients – that was what we called them – or occasionally 'inmates' – but I suppose both are probably thought politically incorrect nowadays. If there was any milk left over it was sent to another hospital nearby. I remember trying to milk a cow by hand.

From The Second World War Until The Early 1980s

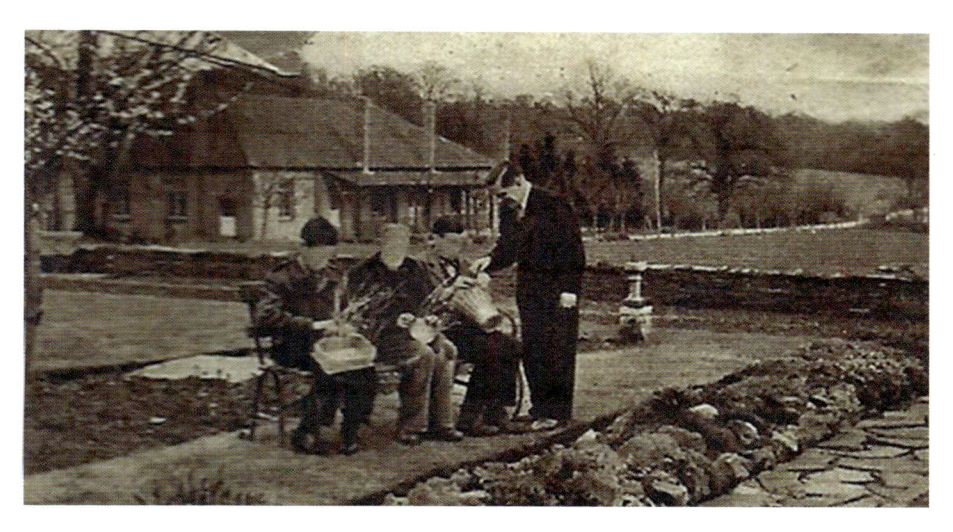

Mr Mason, standing in the gardens with residents.
Photo: The Nursing Mirror, May 1952.

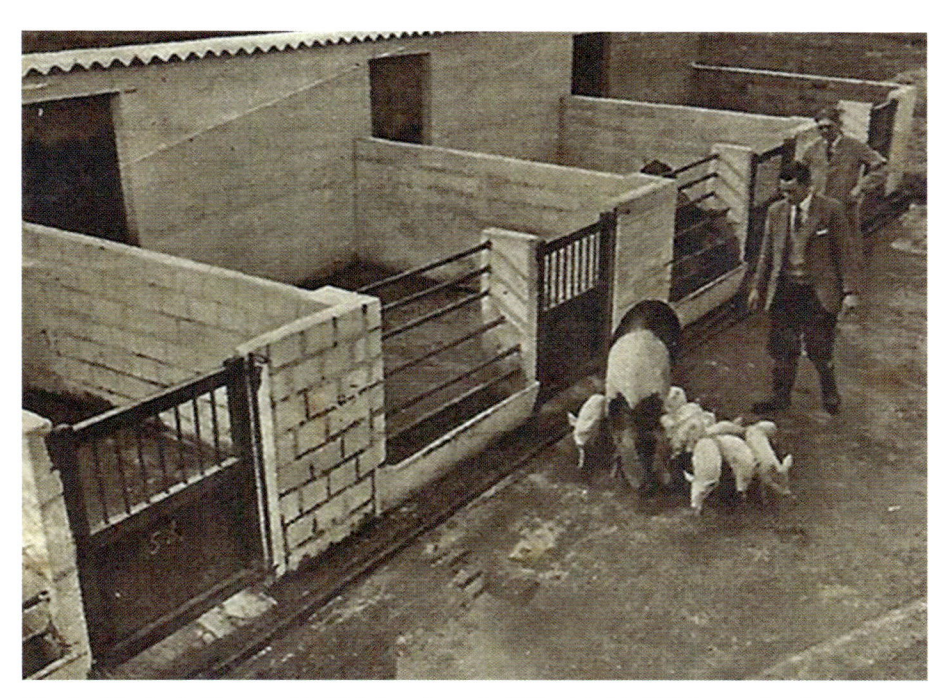

"In the Hygienic Piggery. Mr Hobden, farm bailiff, with Mr T Edgeworth, pigman (background) admire a new litter".
Photo: The Nursing Mirror, May 1952

Most of the 'boys' couldn't really manage it. I had just got the hang of it when the 'boy' who was sitting beside me saw the milk was not going into the pail. So he tried to help but he got a terrible ticking off because he had touched me. The 'boys' looked after the cows under the herdsman, Mr R Moore and they did the mucking out or weeding in the fields or cutting down trees and coppicing. At harvest time they were particularly busy."

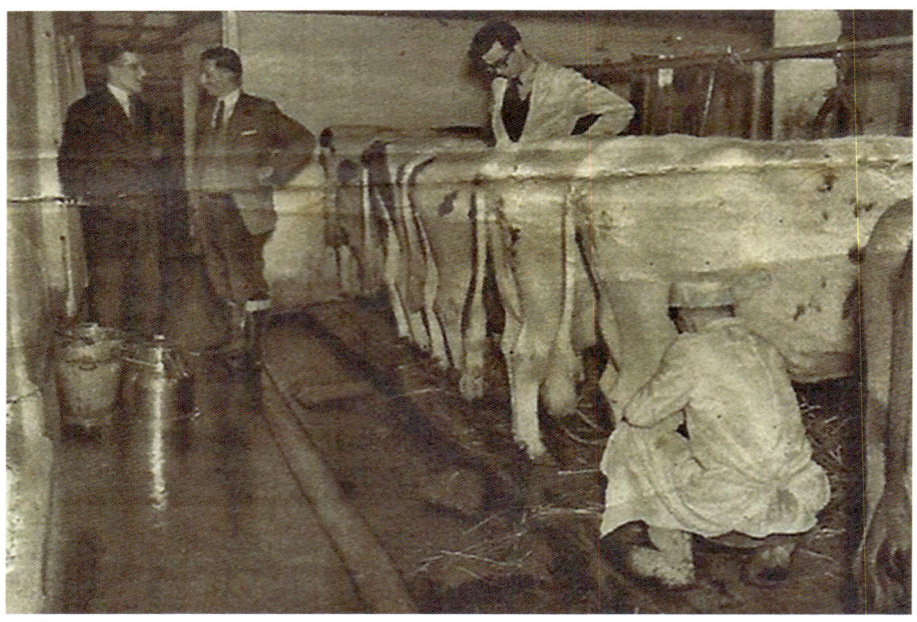

Milking.
Photo: The Nursing Mirror, May 1952

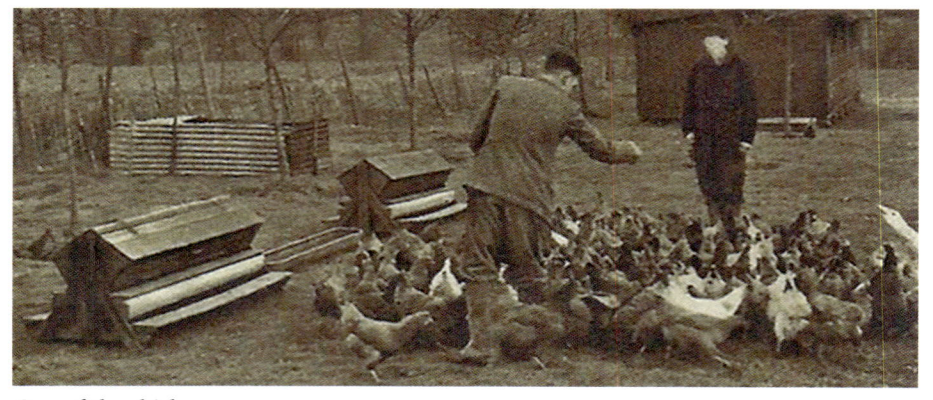

One of the chicken runs.
Photo: The Nursing Mirror, May 1952

From The Second World War Until The Early 1980s

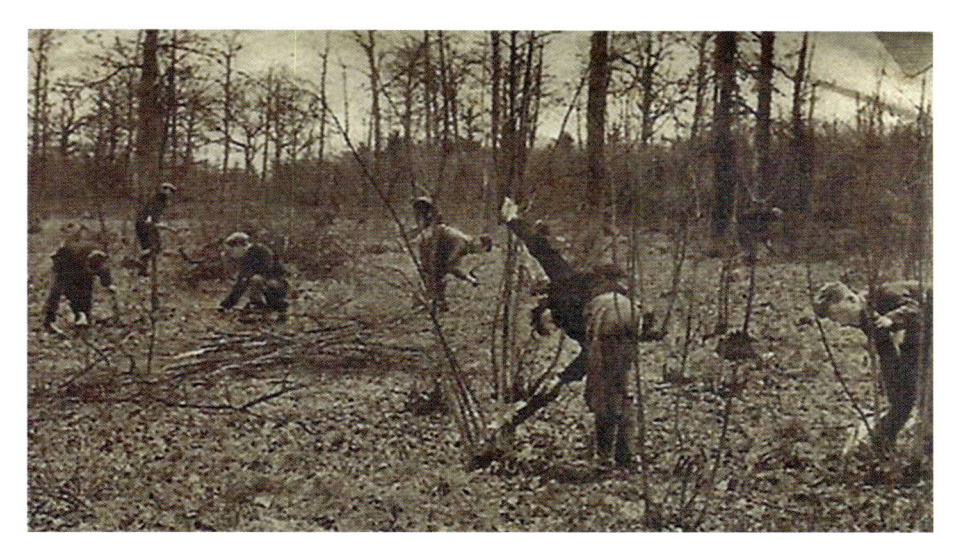

Outdoor Work. Patients busy clearing wooded land.
Photo: The Nursing Mirror, May 1952

The article also provided details of the various houses and 'villas' as the residential buildings were beginning to be called. The Girls' Home apparently housed sixty-eight people but this seems to have included five staff – shown in the picture below.

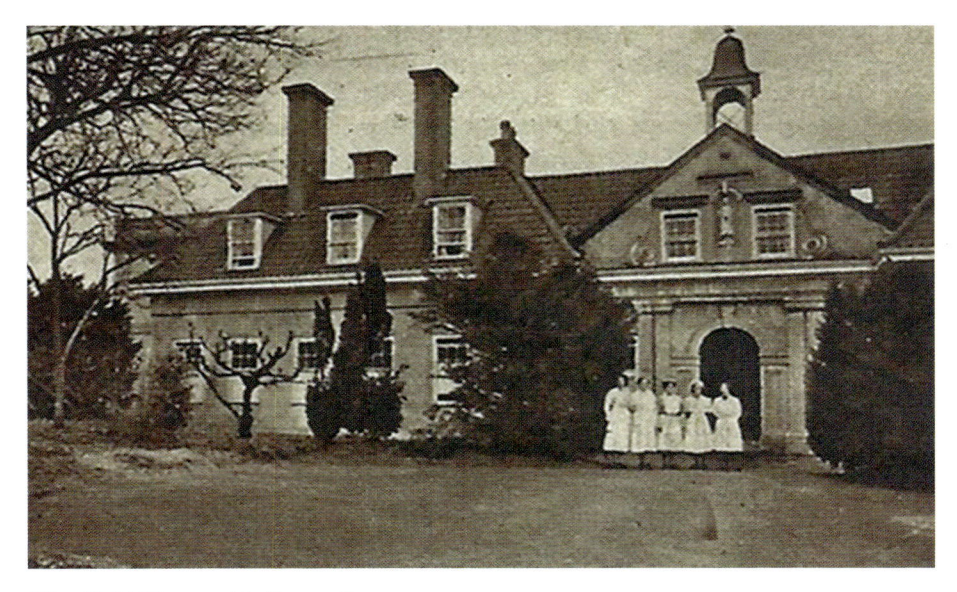

The Girls' House with five staff.
Photo: The Nursing Mirror, May 1952

The Princess Christian Farm Colony and Hospital 1895–1995

There was a description of the laundry work and also details of the sewing undertaken by the 'girls'. The laundry was a large undertaking. It was staffed by twenty-five females, who without any sort of machinery laundered over two thousand five hundred articles per week. Every article was washed by hand, with pressing being done by flat irons which were heated on coke burning stoves. Joy Dolling confirms it was not until the late 1950s or early 1960s that more modern equipment was introduced. "The original method may have been old-fashioned but it provided excellent therapy which gave the patients a feeling of independence and a will for hard work which was very beneficial." The Nursing Mirror article continues with a description of the Sewing Room – sometimes called the Needlework Room – which was also within the Girls' Home. During the daytime it employed about twenty 'girls' under the supervision of a seamstress and an assistant. Joy Dolling adds, "Most of the articles of linen and female attire were made here. In addition, they did repairs. In the evenings an occupational therapy class was held for those wishing to take part; and some really good decorative embroidery and rugs were made." The article goes on to describe the houses for the 'boys'. "The main male block, Trench House, provides living accommodation for thirty-three patients and also includes the kitchen, stores and offices. The Oast House accommodates twenty-three male patients and incorporated a recreation room."

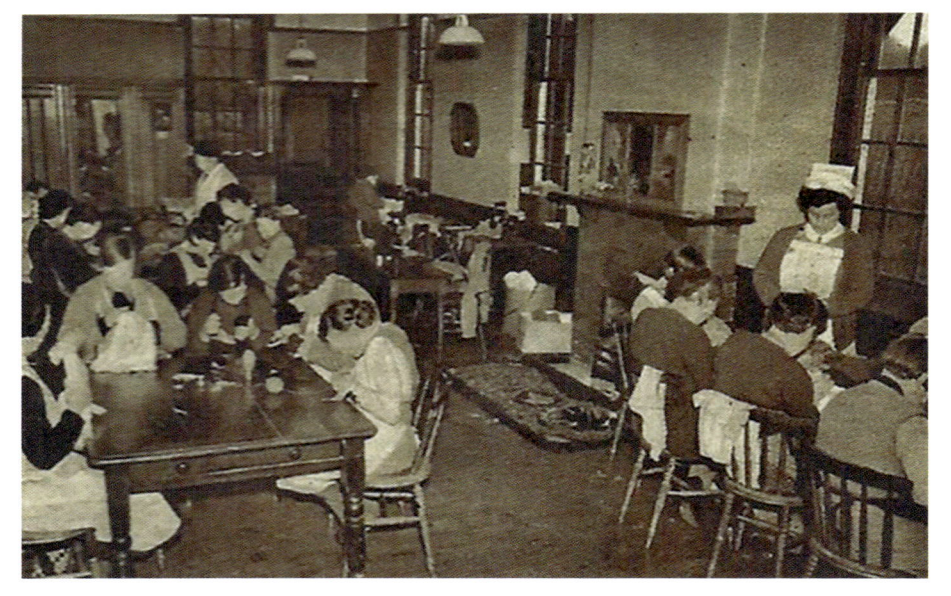

In the Sewing Room 1952.
Photo: The Nursing Mirror, May 1952

From The Second World War Until The Early 1980s

The article has pictures of the 1906/07 Clough Williams-Ellis building with its decorative oast houses at each end but says – wrongly – that it had been used for drying hops in the early 19th century. The Oast House which had originally been bought with the farm had been taken down and a new version rebuilt using the Clough Williams-Ellis design. (The construction of the mid-19th century oast houses was very basic with only four and a half inch walls, and they did not easily adapt to a dwelling.)

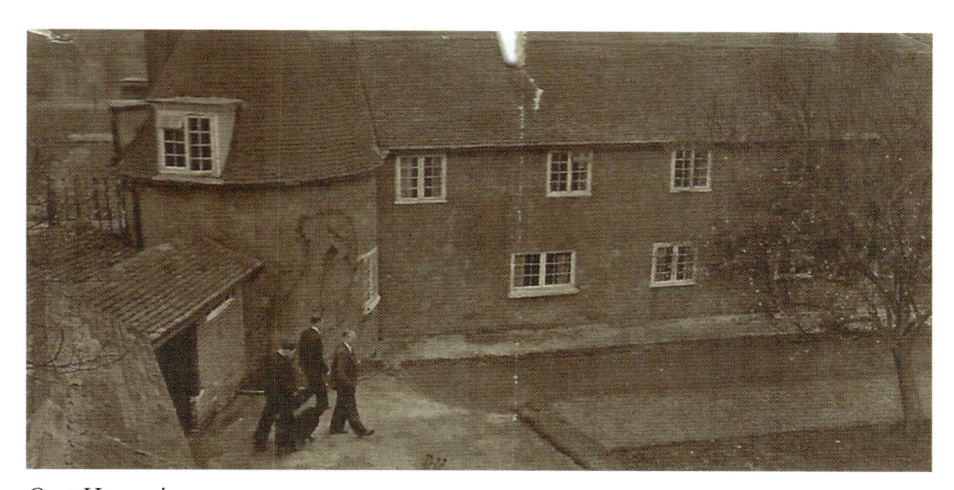

Oast House: in foreground l.to r: Nursing Assistant H Neasham; Chief Nurse E C Mason and Mr S Russell, Superintendent.
Photo: The Nursing Mirror, May 1952

Three Bedroomed Circular Dormitory in the rounded end of the Oast House.
Photo: The Nursing Mirror, May 1952

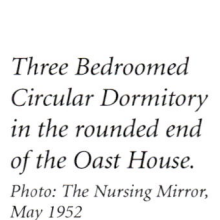

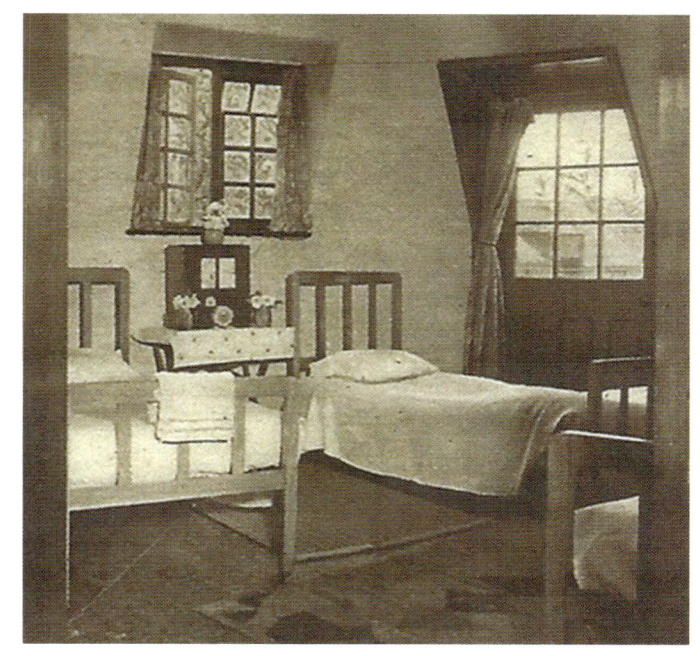

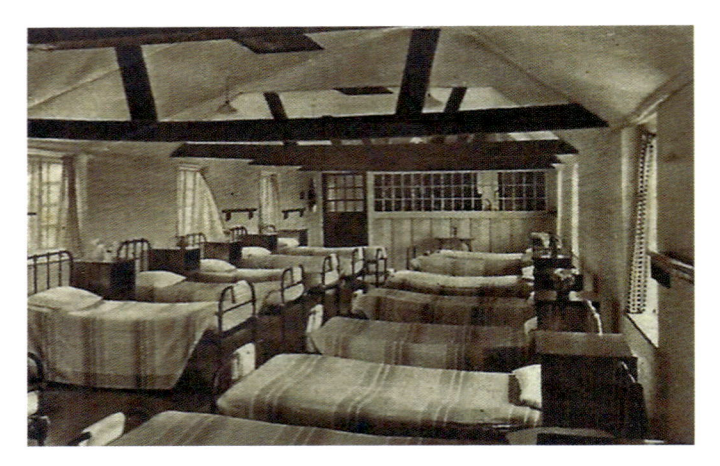

Oast House: The Large Dormitory.
Photo: The Nursing Mirror, May 1952

The next building described is the Farm Villa – the original Upper Hollenden Farmhouse which the article explained was a quarter of a mile down the road from the main buildings. It housed twenty-three patients and staff. The patients were all men. This late 18th century farmhouse, which had beams and oak floors – seen below on the right of the photo – had been extended to include dormitories and a dining room with cooking facilities. In front of the house (to the left of the photograph below) was an orchard.

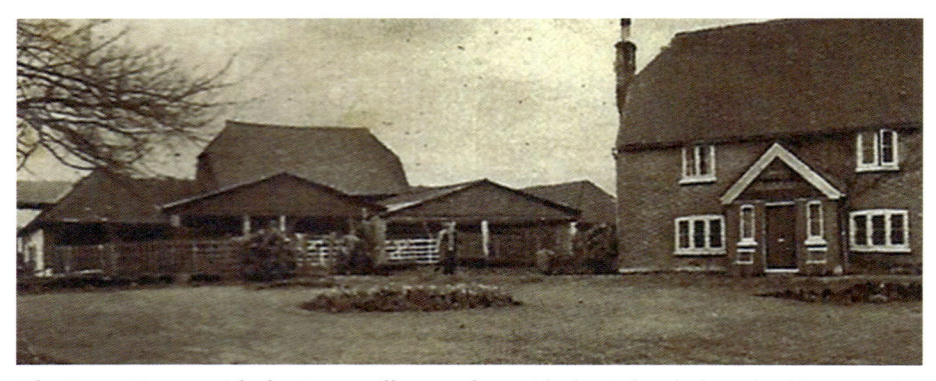

The Farm House, with the Farm Villa, together with the Colony's farm buildings on the left of the photo.
Photo: The Nursing Mirror, May 1952

Further down Riding Lane, past the Farm, was the Cottage Hostel "which housed thirteen patients." The article goes on to say what many people have said. "The Colony was like a big estate and didn't look a bit like a hospital. The houses and villas, including the Girls' Home, were located at distances over the whole estate."

Superintendents and Senior Nursing Officers: 1948-1990

As well as the Farm Manager, there was also the Superintendent who oversaw the running of the many parts of the Hospital itself and – albeit officially under the Leybourne doctors – its medical care. It is not clear whether the Farm Manager reported to the Superintendent. It seems that officially that he must have done; but the two jobs were clearly differentiated and one guesses that a sensible Superintendent was more than happy to let the Farm Manager get on with his side of the Colony. Robin Ballard remembers a number of the men who had the Superintendent's role in the forty years after the War. Some local people say that a Mr Ryall was appointed to run Princess Christian when the Health Service took over, replacing the long-serving Miss Pitman. However, the previously quoted Nursing Mirror article from 1952 reports that the Superintendent was Mr S Russell. So seemingly, Mr Russell had preceded Mr Ryall. Following them was Mr Ed Mason who had joined the Hospital staff in 1950 as the Chief Male Nurse before being promoted in 1959. Fairly soon afterwards, he was succeeded by Mr Joe Kenyon. Robin Ballard remembers Mr Kenyon as "a jolly chap: he was brought up in the North of England and was anxious to open up the Hospital more – to let the public see what the Hospital was like. He was very keen on sport too. There were cricket matches with celebrities. I remember one against some jockeys." Another man who lived locally, Bob Duffin, knew Joe Kenyon well and was involved with the cricket matches in his capacity as Captain of Hildenborough Cricket Club. "Joe had come from working in a hospital in Bristol. He was a small bloke, very physical, thick set, bushy eyebrows, and, being a Lancashire man, he had a strong Lancashire accent and was friendly with absolutely everybody. There's a photo of him in the Hildenborough Village Hall." (In fact, the photo in the Village Hall turns out to be a long-serving Hildenborough school master, not Joe Kenyon. So, while there must have been similarities between the two men, the photograph has not been included). "He treated all the patients – the 'boys' and 'girls' – as friends and he very much wanted to integrate Princess Christian into the community as far as possible. He encouraged local people to join in with all sorts of things. As well as informal dances and gatherings which took place regularly, Joe introduced more official dances which the public were encouraged to come to – and they were almost always sold out. There was one around New Year and three others spread over the year. The most famous event was when Joe got a friend, Mick Channon, involved. Mick had been a nationally known footballer, playing for Southampton and, when he retired, he'd become a racehorse trainer. Mick knew lots of film stars and jockeys and Joe persuaded him to get a team together for a celebrity cricket match against the Hildenborough Cricket Club. So, as Captain, I became very involved. It was a wonderful occasion and, I guess, got Joe a good amount of extra money for the Colony. But, most importantly, it got everyone locally more involved, which was what Joe wanted. He was a lovely man and a very close friend." Ralph Cooke, husband of the long-serving Administrator, Marion Cooke, has extra memories of the match. "Marion and I had got to know Joe very well. As everyone says, he was a wonderful chap – always very lively and cheerful. He had played professional football for Accrington Stanley and had also been a professional cricketer. One or maybe two times there were big charity cricket matches and I remember a jockey's team organized by the well known National Hunt rider, Josh Gifford, playing against an actors' team organized by, I think it was Edward da Sousa. The match really did get huge crowds." Another local explained yet another aspect of the cricket match. It was Nurse Ursula Taylor who was the person who knew Edward de Sousa and it was she who arranged for him to get involved.

The Cricket Club helped to increase understanding between the village and the Colony. As we have seen, for a good number of years one of the 'boys', Derek Bance, was the Club's scorer. Ian Cowdray, who was brought up in Hildenborough in the late 1960s and played cricket for Hildenborough, says, "I remember Joe Kenyon but there was also a 'resident' who came with him. Although the man walked a bit like Charlie Chaplin, he was one of our best batsmen. So the Club as a whole certainly helped build a link between the Colony and the people who lived nearby. I was also in the Hildenborough Youth Club and we used to go along to the dances at P.C. At first it was a bit scary. Some of the people there were badly disfigured, but because I had sort of grown up with Princess Christian people all around me, I probably wasn't as afraid as I would have been otherwise."

Robin Ballard continues, "Around 1972 Mr Kenyon retired as Superintendent and Mr Bell [Jim] took over. Because of the developing, more modern style of medical care, his title became Senior Nursing Officer, rather than Superintendent. Mr Bell was Scottish. He did away with the old army type of uniforms the men had worn when they worked at the Farm and they were allowed more freedom to wear what they liked. He brought even more openness and there was now a psychologist who came in about twice a week from Leybourne." One local remembers the clinical psychologist as Peter Anger, who had escaped from Czechoslovakia under a lorry. "He was a lovely man and we all used to laugh that a psychologist was called 'anger' – not what you'd want." Robin Ballard adds, "Some of the 'boys' and 'girls' were not really ill and it would have been possible to let them live out in the community. Others needed various types of medical help which was provided either by outside experts from Leybourne or more often by the local GPs." Robin particularly remembers Dr Stanley Davison. "Dr Davison had been one of the main doctors in the Hildenborough and Leigh area since 1937. He took over at Princess Christian from the older Dr Fraser. He was well into his forties at the start of the Second World War, so he was not drafted into the army and was left to run the large practice, as well as looking after the Colony, almost single-handed. He was a lovely man. He was my doctor too – he always had freezing cold hands though. When his son, Guy, was fatally injured in a terrible shooting accident in 1956, they said Dr Davison still felt he had to be in the surgery the next day to look after the patients. Then there was Dr Peter Skinner. He was lovely too." Peter Skinner had joined Dr Davison's practice in 1957 and became the Princess Christian GP from the early 1960s. His son, Adam, who had overseen the gardeners, went on to study medicine and became a local GP in Westerham. To be the GP for the Colony was a time-consuming role, sometimes involving a visit almost every weekday and, when necessary, at weekends. Dr Ken Evans, one of his successors as Senior Partner at the Hildenborough practice, recalls Dr Skinner's dedication. "He used to go to Princess Christian at least twice a week, often more, to look after people and to dispense drugs but he also assessed individual patients with the Leybourne psychiatrists to see if they could be allowed to move more towards the outside world. And because the GP practice gave a 24 hour service in those days, it meant that quite a few of us from the practice – Bill Callum, Brian Glaisher, John Kelynack and myself found ourselves going out at odd hours to help the 'boys' and 'girls' as Peter always used call the men and women there – I think that it was the regular way of describing them." Peter Skinner's widow, Barbara, also remembers those days well. "Sometimes I'd go along with Peter. When we arrived, all the patients would shout 'ello doctor and they'd hug him and dribble all over him. Then they'd dribble all over me too. There was one particularly large man, Lennie, who could turn difficult and violent. But he liked Peter and he used to come and have tea with us at our home in Hildenborough. Once, when Peter and I were in the middle of tea – my mother-in-law was there too – Peter got called away. Lennie arrived and, because Peter wasn't there, he became very agitated. I was fairly worried as my mother-in-law was really frightened. Luckily, before anything too bad happened, Peter came back. Eventually, sometime later, Lennie had so many problems – and caused so many problems – that he had to go back to Leybourne – one of the very few I guess. Peter used to spend hours and hours at Princess Christian and you never really knew when something would come up. I remember once we were driving to a friend's dinner party. We were late as usual – Peter had got called out to someone. Anyway, as we were driving down Riding Lane, we saw two of the 'girls' walking away from Princess Christian with their dolls – wheeling them along in their prams. So we stopped – because they certainly weren't meant to be out that late – and, of course, they were very vulnerable. So we put them in the car and drove them back to Princess Christian. They were thrilled to be in THE DOCTOR'S car – so we were even later for the dinner party. But Peter loved his work at Princess Christian. When he retired, Bill Callum formally took over the role but all of the doctors in the practice got involved."

As has been mentioned, Peter's son, Adam Skinner, worked at Princess Christian for six months or so in the summer of 1975 when he was eighteen and waiting to start his medical training at Guys Hospital. "I had been working as a hospital porter at the Kent & Sussex Hospital in Tunbridge Wells, when I was told that they needed a new head gardener at Princess Christian. So I applied and found myself officially in charge of around a dozen of the 'boys' and responsible for looking after the gardens around Alexander House, Glen House and all the main buildings. There were greenhouses located near Alexander House which produced tomatoes and cucumbers for the Hospital kitchen and one of my 'boys' became very keen on planting long rows of aubergines – although I don't remember whether they matured, let alone whether they were ever used in the kitchen. But I remember the tomatoes that I and the 'boys' had cultivated over many long hours in the greenhouses. They matured magnificently and I proudly took boxes of them to the main kitchen. A few days later, I was very disappointed when I visited the kitchens again to find them rotting away unused. However, the bedding plants that we grew were all used in the flower beds around the various houses. I had a wonderful time. The 'boys' were great and I am still convinced that they had a really good life at Princess Christian. There was only one major incident and I suppose I was officially responsible. For weeks we had been cutting down two or three foot high grass and weeds from the flowerbeds around all the houses. We had piled it into a huge 'hay stack'. The problem arose because one of the 'boys', Ian – who was normally fairly responsible – was a smoker and was allowed matches – the only one who was. Somehow one of the others got hold of the matches and decided to be helpful and light the hay stack. It went up like an inferno. But the snag was that it was rather near the newly built Staff Social Club – which many of the staff and 'boys' had helped to build. We all rushed round with our spades trying to stop it getting to the Social Club. But it wasn't going to work, so we ended up with two or three fire engines. But that was – I'm glad to say – unusual. A normal day would be me cycling up from our house in Hildenborough to Princess Christian and getting my team working. Each one was different, of course, but they were all eager to please – well, there was one who could be difficult – but there was never any risk of danger. At lunch time, I would cycle along to the main Farm building and have something to eat with Jack Clayton, the Manager there and Felix who looked after the poultry. Felix had a great big moustache – and his eggs did get used in the kitchens – not like my tomatoes. The other man I remember was Fred Ayling. He was the staff maintenance man. He was always playing practical jokes and, one day, he let the tyres down on my bike and laughed a lot when he saw my face. I thought that I'd get my own back, so a few days later I took the rotor arm out of his car. When he tried to start it to go home he couldn't get it to fire and he got more and more puzzled. Eventually, I told him. And *we* all laughed quite a lot. On Sundays there was a Church service in the Pitman Hall and nearly all the 'boys' and 'girls' went. I took over playing the organ from my younger brother, Quentin. We played all the happy, straightforward hymns – 'Onward Christian Soldiers', 'If You're Happy and You Know It', and so on. The Chaplain came over from Leybourne Grange. He was very good with them – although there was always a lot of shouting and getting up and walking around." This memory of the Sunday Church services at the Colony is confirmed by people from Hildenborough who remember there was a continuing close relationship between Princess Christian and the various vicars at St John's at Hildenborough.[69] Joy Dolling remembers a man from Princess Christian who used to come to St John's. He loved the hymns and had a particularly powerful voice. "Unfortunately, he couldn't read the words and couldn't sing anything in tune," says Joy. "I remember once – after the man had finished some time after everyone else, the Vicar, Bob Bawtry, said it was lovely to hear 'Fred' in good voice (not his real name: he now lives in Tonbridge) and that he was sure God was listening too and had understood everything the man had sung." Another local couple, Brian and Gillian Taylor, remember the curate in the 1980s, Rev Karl Wiggins, who befriended 'Fred'. Fred regularly came to have tea with him. As curates are moved on to greater things, the time came for Rev Wiggins to leave Hildenborough. There was a farewell service and at the end 'Fred' sat there weeping at the loss of his friend.

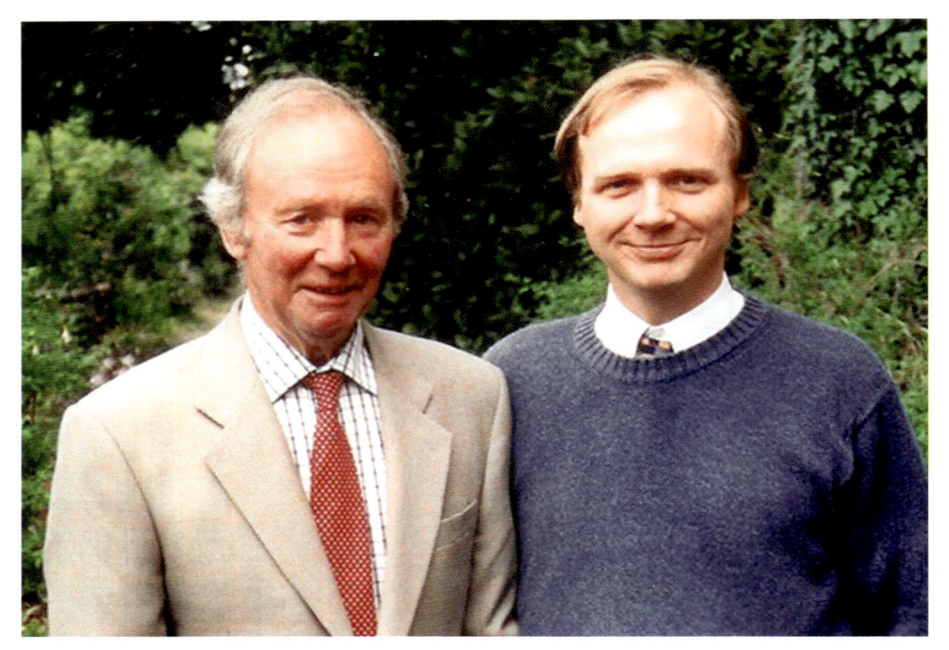

Dr Peter Skinner, the GP who looked after Princess Christian patients from the early 1960s until the mid-1970s, with son Adam, who also helped at the Princess Christian Hospital as a student.

Adam Skinner remembers other aspects of the Hospital's life in the 1970s. "There was the annual sports day. I remember one of the 'boys', Victor Gibb, always used to win the sprints. He was a great hit with the 'girls'. Were there ever problems about sex? I'm not sure: but it would have been likely. The 'boys' and 'girls' would have had all the natural instincts. So maybe 'why not?' But I don't know."

In the mid-1970s, after more than fifteen years as the Princess Christian GP, Adam's father, Dr Peter Skinner retired and the late Dr Bill Callum, again from the Hildenborough practice, became the main GP. However, as we have seen, sometimes other GPs from the practice had to go to look after the patients at Princess Christian and Dr Ken Evans, together with his wife, Ann, remembers well the occasional eccentricity of the normally gentle and friendly patients. Dr Evans expands on the role GPs had. "Until 1948 Princess Christian was separately managed as a charity. Only in 1949 or 1950, when the NHS officially took it over, did it become a subsidiary to Leybourne Grange, with main medical direction from Leybourne. Patients came from all over the South East: it was not just for people in the Sevenoaks or Tonbridge areas." [Although there were a few 'patients' or 'colonists' from the local area, it does not seem relevant to give specific names. However, the families of these people have said how grateful they were for the care given to their children.]

By the 1980s, while the consultant psychiatrists from Leybourne seemed to have formally visited Princess Christian only two or three times a year,[70] the day-to-day doctoring continued to be done by the local GPs. The work involved everything from sore throats to appendices. "The patients at Princess Christian were by no means all Down's syndrome," continues Ken Evans. "There was a wide range of causes and symptoms for what the Victorians had called 'feeble-mindedness' and what we today would call 'being on the autistic spectrum'. Even when I was a medical student in the late 1950s, there were formal classifications and terms which we'd blanch at twenty years later. The ones I remember were 'imbecile', as well as 'mongol', but there was a range of others. They gradually got changed – usually for the better. But eventually the terms became less specific, more politically correct – but sometimes less useful! Thinking back over the fifty years since I qualified, I have seen big changes in the treatment of the whole wide range of the mentally ill. I remember when families used to be very ashamed if they had a relative with learning disabilities. Now this is not really the case. The new drug treatments undoubtedly helped make it possible to have more men and women of the type who lived at Princess Christian moved into the community; but, in reality, the kind of people who were sent to Princess Christian were not usually disturbed enough to need any drugs. Eventually, several of the staff houses in Riding Lane were converted into 'hostels' or 'villas' for residents, who could be moved from the Hospital, and it worked well. For many years the local residents who lived near Princess Christian learnt to be fond of its patients; and it's good to see that attitudes to those with the various types of learning disabilities have changed for the better. In the 1930s and 1940s, and I remember much later even in the 1950s and 1960s, to have a backward child could often break up a family. It is great to see that society has become more understanding – even if the strain on families having to cope at home with a child with difficulties will continue – however much help and understanding there is."

Life for the 'Boys' and 'Girls' in the 1960s

Joy Dolling has further memories of her childhood in Hildenborough in the late 1950s and early 1960s. "Most of the patients, once told what and how to do things, needed very little supervision both in their day work and recreationally. Many of them would carry on with basket making, table mat making, rug making, wood carving and needlework in their spare time. They all seemed very happy and enjoyed what they were doing. Mr Mason, the Superintendent and a close friend of our family, collected old clocks and watches and some of the men worked on them and restored them to working order. The patients also took part in a variety of sports and outdoor pastimes. In the winter there was football. The patients played both home and away matches against other 'Colonies' and outside teams. Indoors, there was table tennis, billiards and snooker, bagatelle, darts and many other games, such as cribbage, draughts, dominoes, etc. It was particularly noticeable how popular jig-saw puzzles were, especially among the less able patients. There was a cinema show once a week and dances on occasions. During the summer months there were many outdoor sports, such as cricket, tennis, putting, rounders, stool ball, quoits, skittles and netball. Occasionally mixed games were organized but they had to be supervised. The Annual Sports Day was held on the August Bank Holiday. Concerts were arranged at intervals and a Colony Orchestra was formed from patients and staff. In most of the recreations, a competitive spirit was encouraged and tournaments with suitable handicaps took place. As the Colony was in a country setting, many of the purely rural sports were possible. In the 1940s and 1950s small parties of boys were allowed to go 'rabbiting' and in the autumn a number of them would act as beaters for outside shooting parties, the resultant birds being consumed by the patients and staff. Many of the patients were given their own plot of land and made really good garden displays. Prizes were given once a year for the best gardens. Tobacco was a very popular plant and some quite good results were obtained for the end product. This, of course, would not be allowed today! When in season, several patients were allowed to go searching for mushrooms in the early morning and it was amusing to see the look of triumph when a good haul was produced. As far as possible, the patients at the Colony lived in conditions that were like normal homes. At least thirty to forty of the patients were allowed out without supervision. They had to be back for tea or supper. Some of the less able were taken shopping in Tonbridge. Some came to our Church. They were part of our Hildenborough community. All were welcomed by the villagers and their disabilities were ignored. I know that our family and many others in the locality applauded the work and care that went on at the Colony for those who were less able than the majority."

Clearly, the 'patients' were kept cheerful and busy and, indeed, *kept themselves* busy and cheerful. From virtually every report we have, the staff did an excellent job and the community accepted the men and women from the Colony as a normal part of their life. What was only just beginning to happen in a formal way, however, was the thought that potentially a good number of the men and women could actually live in the outside world. This was only really actively beginning to be talked about in the 1970s.

Farm Managers

The Farm at Princess Christian had continued to operate during the Second World War, although seemingly on a reduced basis. From the 1940s or even just before the War until the early 1960s, as we have heard, the Farm Manager was Mr W Hobden who lived at Brownway Cottage, Riding Lane. The farm had a tractor and the tractor driver, Fred Gardener – known as 'Garnie' – who lived next door to Mr Hobden.

Mr Hobden was succeeded as Farm Manager in the early 1960s by Mr R Palmer, who lived in Underriver. Robin Ballard remembers him as a big strong man who had lost his left arm in a tractor accident when he was a young man. "He could drive a manual car or the tractor with ease and when it came to hay-making he could pitch a bale of hay onto a loaded trailer with just his right arm." Another tractor driver, who probably succeeded Fred Gardener, was Don Perrin who lived in Church Road, Hildenborough. He worked at the farm for many years until his retirement. The next Farm Manager was Mr John Clayton – usually known as Jack – who succeeded Mr Palmer in the 1980s and who was there until the Hospital closed. He lived at Chestnuts, a Princess Christian house, in Vines Lane before moving to Tonbridge.

The role of Farm Manager involved two very different skills – and it needed a special person to combine the two. Firstly, the person had to be an experienced farmer; and, secondly, he had to be able to handle the patients who came with a reasonably wide range of ability and their own very personal outlooks. Some could be lazy, others keen to work; some were quiet and would do what they were asked but others could become aggressive if they felt that they were being thwarted or belittled. It was never a straightforward job.

Problems with the Weather

The Farm and the Colony as a whole had not only the normal eccentricities of the British weather with which to contend but there were a variety of one-off weather problems. Seemingly, everyone coped well. The winter of 1962/63 was very long and severe. Robin Ballard remembers Riding Lane being blocked by snow drifts which were as high as the hedges. It was a difficult time for Princess Christian, trying to keep everything working in such low temperatures and, often in winter, frozen pipes were a regular problem. The cattle had to be kept under cover to protect them from the cold. Quite a few nursing staff remained at the hospital overnight when there was snow, rather than risk not being able to get to work the following day. One thing Robin Ballard will never forget was the thousands of hungry wood pigeons that decimated the kale one year which had been growing in the field in front of Alexander House. "The crop was intended to be winter feed for the cattle but it was frozen solid and the leaves were almost the only greenery visible above the snow – apart from the pigeons! In the end, a shoot was organized and hundreds of pigeons were killed in a bid to try to save the crop. There was more freak weather in September 1968. This time heavy rain badly flooded large parts of Hildenborough and Tonbridge. Princess Christian itself was lucky not to be affected by flood water getting into the buildings but the drive leading up to Girls' Home was impassable for quite a distance where the Hilden Brook burst its banks. Also, the chicken unit situated on the other side of the road bridge, up to the Girls' Home, was flooded by water cascading along the drive from high ground opposite the Girls' Home. Riding Lane was flooded beside the recreation ground down towards Hildenborough and was a raging torrent at Club Cottages making the road impassable. It was also flooded at Stone Cottages near to the end of Riding Lane. Vines Lane, too, was flooded by the stream that feeds the lake at The Vines, with fast moving water flowing through the woods on one side of the road and across the fields further down from Chestnuts. Mill Lane was also flooded in several places leaving Princess Christian (or PCH as it was often called by then) and neighbouring properties virtually cut off for much of the Sunday."

When there was very heavy snow in December 1984 which virtually cut off Princess Christian, the staff made huge efforts to get to the site and keep things going. W. Cowell, the Director of Nursing Services at Leybourne, wrote a public note saying, "a short thank you to all staff for the commitment displayed during the recent Arctic conditions… with special thanks to all drivers and night staff."[71]

Developments in the 1970s

We know a fair amount about the advances which were being introduced in the 1970s from a short History of Princess Christian written in May

1981 by Mrs K Hume, a past Chairman of the House Committee, with Mr Roy Cooper, the Senior Nursing Officer in the 1970s. It is particularly valuable to have this assessment from a senior staff member.

1972 saw the introduction of a full-time teacher which meant that a number of residents were able to benefit from educational classes. Additionally, local people with teaching experience used to give lessons to individuals. The wife of the Hildenborough Headmaster, Mary Perry, used to go up to help, together with another local lady, Janet Richardson. There was one 'boy', to whom Janet was explaining simple maths. He was excellent at addition, but he could not – and did not want to – understand subtraction. When Janet set him some simple subtraction questions and then said some of the answers were not really right, he became very upset. Bill Richardson, Janet's husband, explains, "If they felt they were being criticized, they could get very cross. But it was just their way of trying to cope with life." 1972 also saw the formation of Princess Christian's own Multi-Disciplinary Assessment Team – which included the local GP. Over the coming two years every hospital resident was evaluated by this team of experts so that an individual plan was worked out for every patient.

In 1973 two bungalows were built in the grounds of Alexander House which became home for five men in one and five women in the other. The idea was to encourage them to live with suitable help in what would be 'family conditions' and to prepare at least some of them to live in the wider world, if the opportunity arose. One such opportunity did indeed arise the following year when the Hospital was offered what was called a Group Home in Tonbridge and four men moved there. In 1974 a new hut was purchased for the Occupational Therapy Department. This not only gave more space but meant that there could be an increase in the variety of activities undertaken. 'Industrial Therapy' was also introduced. And with the acquisition of a spacious bathroom in a nearby building, self-help teaching programmes about personal hygiene were also possible. Around this time, the Hospital also acquired the services of a more regular Psychologist as part of the team. Behaviour Modification programmes were introduced including a new intensive programme which met with a fair measure of success. The scheme put certain patients together in what were called Hyper Kinetic Groups. The general teaching, which had been started in 1972, had been expanded. Mr Cooper continues: "By 1981 there were two part-time teachers who gave daily classes, with further ones on three evenings a week for those unable to attend the classes in the daytime because they had outside employment or other activities."

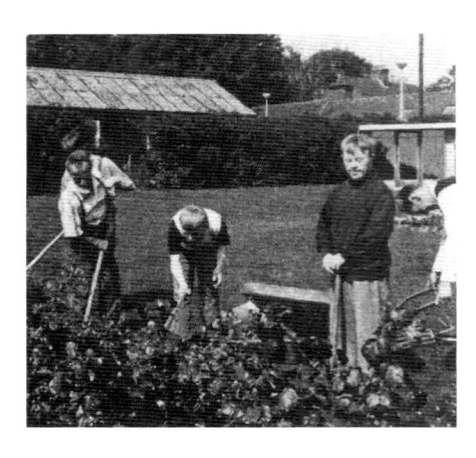

"Every Little Helps"
From Spotlight In-House Magazine Autumn 1978

Mr Cooper's improvements were professional and must have been beneficial. What his account does not mention were the wider changes which were being planned by government and senior civil servants. A flavour of these reforms comes from the minutes of a Leybourne Grange Management Meeting which has survived in the Kent Archive.[72] The Minutes from 24 February 1975 record a meeting with senior DHSS – not NHS – civil servants who make it clear that mental health hospitals, such as Leybourne, must, in the short term, aim to have smaller and less formal units within the institutions; and that, long term, the institutions themselves will be replaced by much smaller, community-based services and buildings. However, the Minutes make no mention of the developments that had been happening at Princess Christian, where a good number of the changes being proposed by the DHSS were already in place or were being planned – if and when money allowed.

Medical Treatments and Nursing in the 1970s and the early 1980s

By the 1970s and the 1980s, the medical care of the Princess Christian residents came in various ways. As we have seen earlier, Leybourne Grange Hospital was theoretically in overall charge and was meant to provide experts. However, it seems from some evidence that Leybourne did not always provide clear or competent leadership and, at least for some periods, their experts do not seem to have been very evident at Princess Christian. The day-to-day care at the Hospital was overseen by the Senior Nursing Officer, who for a good many years in this period was Mr Roy Cooper – the author of the short history described above. Working with him and his staff of nurses and auxiliary nurses was the team of Hildenborough GPs. Dr Ken Evans mentions the medical advances – particularly with drugs – which became available to help those at Princess Christian during the 1960s to 1980s. "The first big breakthrough in care for those who were called mentally sub-normal came in the later 1950s and 1960s. There was a range of new drugs. First were the major tranquillisers, the phenothiazines, such as Largactil and Thorazine. Another was Stelazine, presented as little blue pills which were easy to swallow and which were made locally at the old Tonbridge Gunpowder Mills site. They were used on some patients at Princess Christian but not that many. There were occasional side effects – particularly if the dose was high – such as tremors or anxiety – but the disadvantages were much outweighed by the benefits. A bit later there was another group of drugs – the tricyclic group of drugs such as Tofranil, Surmontil and Anafranil for patients who were depressed. Then later still were the benzodiazipines such as Librium and Valium which were used to keep patients calmer when necessary. There were also a variety of new drugs to help people who had epileptic fits which had fewer side effects than the earlier drugs – although there were only a few at Princess Christian who were epileptics."

There was a separate type of advance concerning drugs in this period. Dr John Ford, formerly the senior partner in another large Tonbridge medical practice, Warders, and a medical historian, explains. "One of the major problems with drugs was getting the patients to keep on taking them when they were meant to. It still is a problem for many people. The breakthrough came in the 1980s with the development of slow-release preparations which could be given by injection into the backside whose action lasted for a month. Modecate and Depixol were those most commonly used. These drugs were used primarily for patients with schizophrenia, so I suspect that not many of these drugs were needed at Princess Christian." However, one example of how this treatment could revolutionize a life came from a daughter – herself a mental health nurse. Her mother was schizophrenic. "It was terrible. On one day she would be fine and the next completely out of her mind and uncontrollable. We kept having to get her sectioned. Then she would be sent to Barming Hospital which was an awful place. This went on for fifteen years. It put a terrible strain on the family – although my children were wonderful. They loved their granny and used to go to Barming quite often when she was sent there yet again. But, when the slow release drugs came along, everything changed and she spent the last fifteen years at home perfectly normal in every way."

The Princess Christian Farm Colony and Hospital 1895–1995

One of the most senior nurses, for many years in charge of the Girls' Home, was Nan Connor. "I had trained as a psychiatric nurse in Dumfries. Then I got married and came to live in Tonbridge. My first job was over at Maidstone in the old Barming Hospital as a Deputy Ward Sister. It was a ghastly place – it hadn't changed much since Victorian times. Then I had a baby – Nina – and, when Nina was very little, I saw an advertisement for a nursing assistant at Princess Christian. It was much nearer home and I hoped, if I got the job, that I could fit the work more easily around the baby. So I went to the interview – it was 1959 – and I wasn't given the Nursing Assistant job – I was offered a job as Acting/Part-time Charge Nurse at the Girls' Home, as it was called at the time. I was there for twenty-nine years, working my way up to full-time Charge Nurse, then Deputy Ward Sister, then to Ward Sister. Eventually – they kept changing titles – I became Ward Manager for the last five years until the Girls' Home, which became known as Glen House, was wound down." Nan remembers the drugs that the doctors prescribed and that they then gave to the 'girls' and the 'boys'.

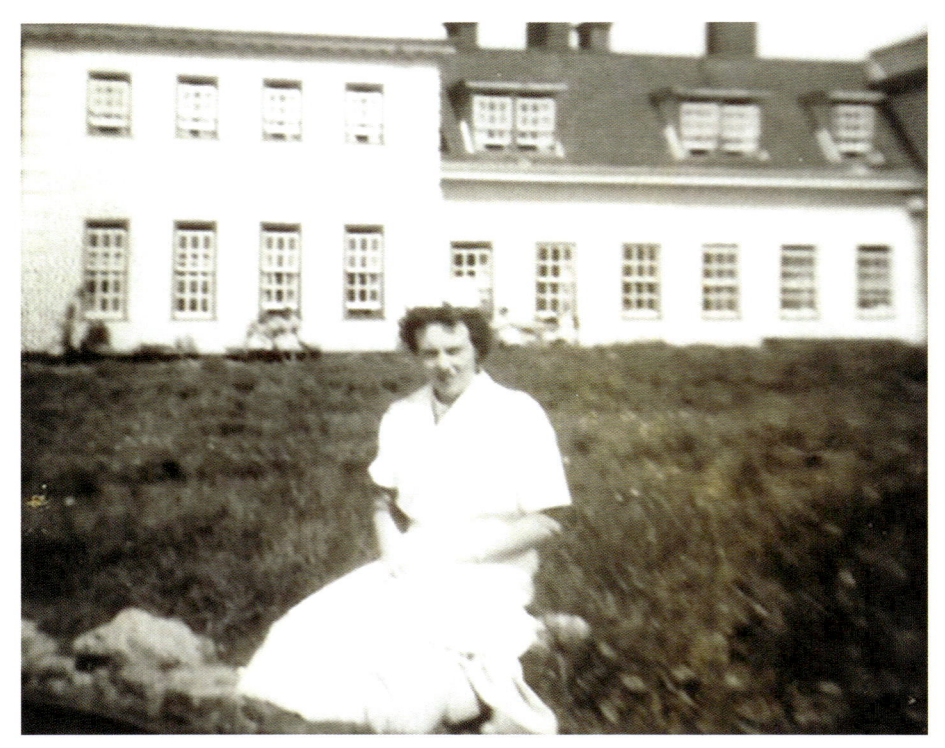

Nan Connor in 1959 sitting on the grass at the back of the Girls' Home.
Photo: from Nan Connor

From The Second World War Until The Early 1980s

"Probably a quarter of the people at Princess Christian were on some kind of pills at any one time. Of course, some were just medicines for ordinary, everyday things but quite a few of the drugs mentioned by Dr Ken Evans and Dr Ford were given out on a routine basis as prescribed by the doctors – although the doses were reviewed every month. Every resident had his/her own drug chart which was scrupulously kept up-to-date every day. In the early years, I remember we had Largactil, Thorazine and Stelazine; then later there was Tofranil and certainly Librium and Valium were prescribed in the 1980s. With regard to epilepsy, the accepted figure nowadays is that one in five people with learning disabilities suffers from some form of epilepsy and that was probably the ratio at Princess Christian. The drugs for epilepsy were useful for most of the people but for the most severe cases, the 'boys' or occasionally the ' girls' would wear protective helmets, so that if and when they fell down, they did not hurt themselves too badly." One nurse mentioned that she still sees some of the patients she remembers from Princess Christian in Tonbridge today and they continue to wear the same padded headgear.

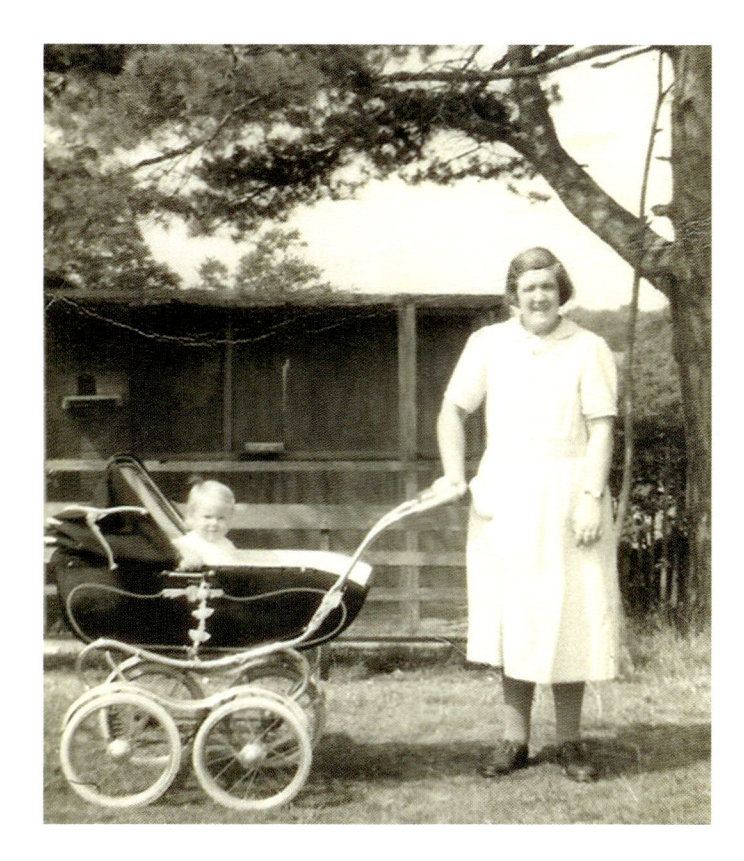

Nina Connor in her pram c. 1960 with Kathleen Chaplin who often looked after Nina as well as her real job of overseeing the kitchen at Glen House.
Photo: from Nan Connor

"Over all the years, the staff I had were all – nearly all – wonderful", says Nan. "And, although some of the younger ones moved on – quite naturally – lots of the older staff stayed for years and years. They were really dedicated and they loved the place. I remember when I first arrived at the Girls' Home that there was a Nurse Black. She lived in Sevenoaks and every day she caught the bus from Sevenoaks to Hildenborough and then walked up to the Hospital – even in the rain or snow – it must be two miles. I've given you the names of lots of the staff I remember. [See Appendix 5]. I still see quite a few of them – it really was like a family. When we first arrived, we were really lucky. The Farm House was available, so the three of us, my husband, Nina and I, were able to move in. We had to pay for it, of course. All staff living in did. It was fifteen shillings a week to start with. Eventually, it was eighteen shillings a week. At this time the Colony had sixty-eight 'girls' and a hundred and forty-seven men. So there were around two hundred and fifteen people for us to look after. I think that it was the most residents there ever was at Princess Christian and I seem to remember that we had a period when we did not take in anyone extra with the aim to get the number down to around a hundred and sixty.[73] When I first arrived the beds in the Girls' Home dormitories were really crammed together – there was hardly room to get between the beds or down the middle of the room. To look after them, we had a Ward Sister and Deputy Ward Sister who lived out and three other staff who lived in, who were expected to deal with any problems overnight – overnight was 8pm to 7am. It was only later that we got staff whose job it was to look after things overnight – although for an interim period we had a night watchman who walked around the outside of all the different buildings. Lots of things changed over the years. When I arrived, the 'girls' lives were fairly regimented. They got up at eight and had their breakfast – which they made for themselves. In fact, they did everything for themselves where they were able to do so – the washing and the laundry which they did it for the whole of P.C. – and the cleaning. The men had to look after themselves too – in those days there were virtually no domestic staff. If the 'girls' weren't doing anything else like the laundry, they'd work in the sewing room where we had two ladies who came in to help and to teach. At one stage, Bob Ballard's wife came to help too. The 'girls' would be there from 9am to mid-day. Then there was a break to get lunch ready and to eat it. Then at 1.15pm, they all went out for a walk until 2pm when it was back to the laundry or in the sewing room until 4pm unless they had other jobs. Bedtime was 8pm when it was a proper lights out. So, as I said, it was fairly regimented, even if there were a few evening rate the Pitman Hall for the church service. (A bridle path went right through the main bit of Princess Christian and past Glen House but the riders had to get off and walk their horses through our grounds.)

"It was always difficult to get suitable work for the residents to do – apart, of course, from the Farm for the 'boys' and the laundry for the 'girls'. In my time, some of the 'boys' were taught bricklaying and a bit of carpentry and at one time we had an upholstery group. And for a time the 'boys' in particular used to assemble plastic toys for a firm in Tonbridge. We really did try to train up the residents for the outside world where possible but it was very rare for a man or a woman actually to leave Princess Christian altogether. There was one man I remember who had done some outside work and got himself a job with the local council cutting the grass. He went to live with a lady in Tonbridge. Another man used to go out each day to the saw mill at Plaxtol and another man used to do gardening locally with a supervisor. Some of the 'girls' used to do outside cleaning jobs. I had one who came to help me at home once a week and one of the 'boys', Tony Sadler, did a milk round. Perhaps the most unusual job was when one of the 'boys' went up regularly to the Cazalet family at Fairlawne in Shipbourne and learned to be a butler. And a 'girl' went too and learned to be a lady's maid. Her big day came when Princess Margaret visited and stayed the night. The next morning Princess Margaret gave our 'girl' a ten shilling note as a tip. That certainly got talked about!"

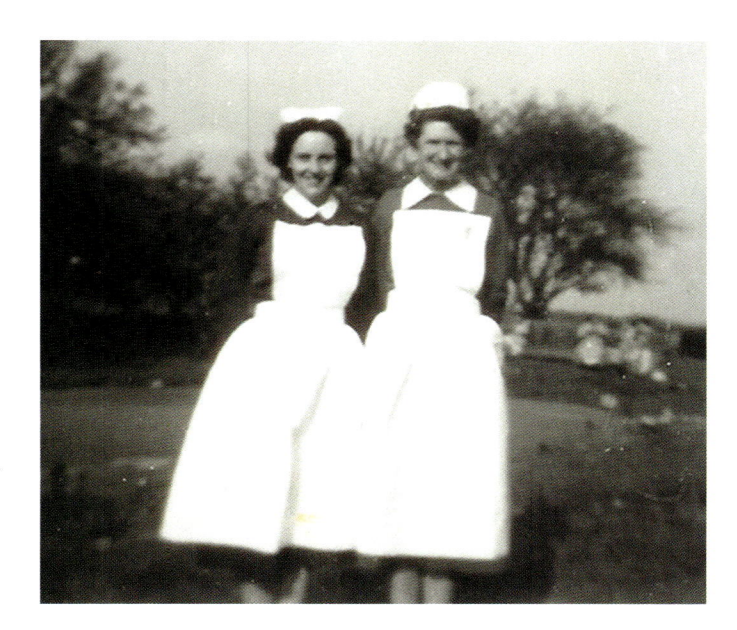

Nurse Nan Connor (on left) with Nurse Dobell in the mid 1960s.
Photo: from NanConnor

Sir Edward Cazalet, when asked recently about these two helpers from Princess Christian, remembered them well. "I became good friends with the man whose name was Herbert. He was not really training to be a butler but he worked with our long-serving butler, Bradbrook, and helped in a dozen different ways – quite a character." Nan continues, "One of the other developments I remember was what we called each other and were called by the residents. For years you would only call someone 'Mr Black' or 'Nurse White'. I cannot even remember some of their Christian names even now. But as things progressed, everyone called everyone – or nearly everyone – by their Christian name. And there were some funny times. There was one man who always took all his clothes off when he went to the toilet. One day we were out on a trip and he said that he 'needed to go'. So knowing – or thinking I knew – what would happen, I went with him. There was no one in the Gents and, as ever, he took all his clothes off. Unfortunately, at that point a man came in, saw my chap – naked – saw me and started to say something. I just said, 'Don't worry: it's one of the perks of the job'. He fled.

"You asked what happened when one of the residents died. There was a proper funeral. Groombridges, the local family undertaker, always did it. There was a service, with flowers and everything and the minister from Leybourne came. If there were family, they were involved; but if there weren't any relatives – quite often the case – the staff and friends from PC were there. Then, after the service, we went to the Crematorium.

"So by 1990/91 'Care in the Community' had really arrived and all my 'girls' from Glen House had gradually been found places to live. Although over the years I still see some of our 'boys' and 'girls' around, I have never felt I ought to ask them – particularly my Glen House 'girls' if they are happy – or happier than they had been when they were with us – our big family. I spent the last year or two as the Ward Manager at the Oast until Princess Christian was finally wound up."

Another nursing sister was the late Mary Beach from Leigh whose husband, John, has provided these recollections of Mary's work. "Mary had been a senior nurse in various general hospitals for a good number of years and had ended up in the Premature Baby Unit at Pembury. She retired when we had children but she knew Dr Peter Skinner well. And when our children went to school, Peter mentioned that an extra nurse was needed at Princess Christian. So from 1977 until 1988, Mary was one of the three main nurses at Princess Christian. Initially, the job involved helping the two existing Nursing Sisters – both of whom had always specialized in mental health – who could not really cover the 12-14 hour days, seven days a week,

From The Second World War Until The Early 1980s

let alone holidays or when one of them was off sick. In particular, Mary used to do a good number of Saturdays and Sundays from 7am to 8pm, leaving me to look after the children." John recalls that the patients – the 'boys' and 'girls' – were mainly all mentally handicapped, rather than physically handicapped, although there was a wide level and type of disability. Some were quiet; some of the men were very strong and could work at manual jobs for hours; and some could be changeable. John remembers one woman. "She was probably thirty-five. When someone she knew arrived, she would rush and give you a huge bear hug which took your breath away, saying how much she loved you: on another day, you'd arrive and she'd just swear at you – the 'f' word and all the others. There were several whose language was like that but the nurses got used to it. And, of course there were patients who had grown old at Princess Christian and had dementia. Mary mainly worked with the men and women at the main buildings and at Glen House, at the top of the drive but she did not work at Alexander House in Vines Lane. In general her job was similar to a nurse in an old people's home or a disabled person's home and included giving the patients their medicines as prescribed by the doctors, mainly Peter Skinner in those days. She and the other nurses worked mainly under the outside GP, rather than the administration team of Princess Christian. However, in the late 1980s, so many changes were taking place that Mary decided that it was time to leave, although the doctors tried to persuade her to stay."

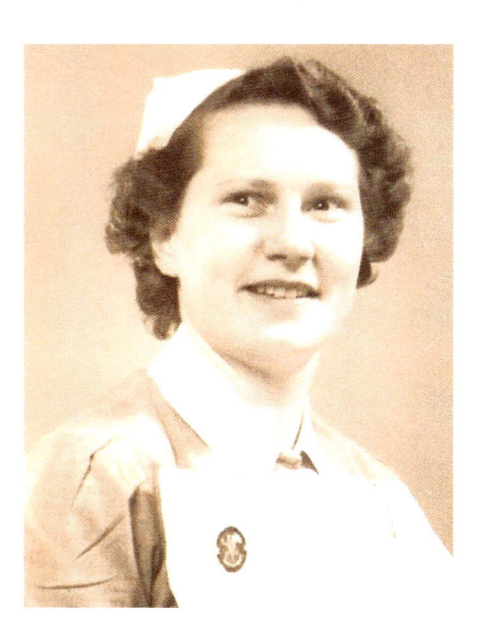

Mary Beach in her nursing sister's uniform c. 1975.
Photo: from John Beach

However, there is another, more detailed description of the day-to-day job of nursing at the Hospital written by a charge nurse, K. K. Fisher, for the house magazine, Spotlight in 1978. His account is given almost in full because it paints such a vivid picture of ordinary life.

A major facet of our Hospital is the Wards. Of course, a hospital ward conjures up row of beds with prostrate people looking sorry for themselves, and in a hushed atmosphere scurrying nurses carrying out their duties of reassuring patients and giving out prescribed treatments. At the end of a relatively short period of time, the nurses see their patients on their feet, leaving Hospital to resume their normal lives once more. But in our Hospital, the ward is the home and possibly the only home many of our patients will ever know. So we refer to our wards as 'Houses' and 'Villas'; i.e. Glen House where our female patients live; and also the Oast House and Alexander House and the Farm Villa with its annex, the Hostel, these last two being for men. We also have two Bungalows – one for males and one for females.

It is sometimes debated who has the hardest and most difficult duties – general nursing or our branch of nursing. Many consider general nursing but I, personally, have never thought so. I have recently spent several weeks as a patient in a general hospital and this experience has confirmed my views. The general nurse has certain specified duties to carry out. She deals with small groups of people who have some insight into what ails them and are co-operative and grateful for the treatment they receive. Yet all nurses have to be tough. For they see people when they are most helpless when even their basic functions have to be seen to and the most gruesome aspects of the human body are seen and dealt with. People have to be lifted, turned, bathed and shaved.

A good nurse has always been the same – cheerful, practical and able to persevere through all difficulties. A nurse has to learn many skills and some knowledge of psychology, like the mental mechanism that makes us tick, helps us to cope with life – such as transference. When a person finds themselves in an unpleasant situation, they put the blame on the Government, their families or God – for to take the blame themselves would be too painful for their minds to accept.

In our branch of nursing, two, three or even one nurse will sometimes find themselves having to cope with 30 to 50 patients. We have not only to deal with the physical and mental welfare of our patients; there are also their private possessions – money, watches, radios, clothing, etc, as well as Hospital property, clothing, etc and including the repairs and checking of the laundry. There are letters to write to relatives and drugs to order. A rough estimation would be that one third of our patients are on some kind of medication.

Nearly all our patients have been with us for years, so we prefer to call our people 'residents'. Their ages range from 20 years to 80 years. I believe there is a project in hand to build a special annex for our senior citizens.

Over the years, you get to know each resident as an individual. I have learnt a lot about myself as well as about them. Some require firmness, others reassurance, coaxing and playful encouragement. They have a routine life which most do not like having to change, for like us all, they are children of habit. It is part of our job to help them acquire good habits as they are not only useful and time-saving but they also make them more socially acceptable.

There are those with behaviour problems which take up a lot of our time. So we have to remember those quiet, passive ones who stay in the background and make contact with them also. This is where our Assessment Meetings prove most useful. The meetings take place on Thursdays when the care nurses from the Wards, along with Nursing Officers, OT Staff and our GP Doctor, discuss each resident and any problems which they may have and how to improve their lives, to occupy, learn and develop. We often conclude that many of our residents do not need full hospital care. But when we examine the alternatives, find that there is nowhere better for them than Princess Christian's Hospital.

I myself would like to apply for a residential place in the new senior citizen's Hostel for when I retire. Laundry, heating, good food, 26in colour television paid for through League of Friends funds (who also provide the Christmas Party), Bonfire night celebrations, Church Services, cinema, discos on Sunday afternoons organized by the V.S.U., and pocket money for town shopping. Dentist every three months, Chiropodist every other week, Dental Hygienist and our good GP Doctor who has never failed to come when asked, day or night, over many years. Summer holidays to the Isle of Wight with Fred Gardner and his band of helpers. Sorry you'll be retired by then as well Fred!

I hope I have been able to communicate to the reader of this article some new and interesting facets about our Hospital. Of course one must remember the other groups of people who help to make the Hospital function – cooks, maintenance men, drivers and last but not least the clerical staff who try to balance the books.

If the staff at the Hospital felt that Princess Christian was a worthwhile place for the residents in the 1970s, the view is echoed by a senior outsider. Dr Malcolm Forsythe was the Medical Officer of Health for Kent 1974-1978 and then the South East Regional Director of the NHS. He remembers Princess Christian well. "It was one of my hospitals but it was a worry-free place. So I didn't have to visit it as often as I had to for the more difficult hospitals. But it was always a pleasure to go round. Peter Skinner was the doctor who looked after it in my day. He was an outstanding GP – the whole practice was excellent in fact. Of course, only the relatively mild cases went to Princess Christian but the quality of life that the residents or in-patients or whatever you'd call them was first rate. It was my people who had to develop suitable places for them to go to when the Hospital was gradually closed down."

Administration

The administration of an organization the size and type of Princess Christian Hospital was a complex task. There were usually over a hundred and fifty residents, all of whom lived and worked in a variety of not very new buildings, many of which needed attention, scattered over a number of sites. There were increasingly complex medical and social provisions, let alone the financial management. In 1973 Marion Cooke, who initially lived in Hildenborough before moving to Leigh, arrived at Princess Christian and for the next twenty-seven years, until 1990, was the Administrator. She says that she thinks of those years as the happiest days of her life. "I got to know all the 'boys' and 'girls' very well; and, even today, when I am shopping in Sainsburys, I'll hear 'Hello Cookie' and one of them will appear. Some of them could be very violent and very abusive but you had to get to understand them and talk them out of their mood in the right way. As well as doing all the office work and organizing the outings, I also ran the shop at Princess Christian. So it was quite a job. My sister, Selma, used to come up to Princess Christian regularly to do the hairdressing." Working with Marion Cooke was Elizabeth Myers. "I was in the office with Marion Cooke for a good number of years. We had a man from Leybourne who was officially the boss – he really did the money side – but we had all the day-to-day organizing and dealings with the men and women. As well as the office work, later on I ran the shop. It was open for an hour in the morning and an hour in the afternoon. The men would be waiting for me to arrive – one always used to be there sitting cross-legged on the ground. Then they would take ages choosing what to buy with their pocket money – it wasn't much. We had sweets and bars of soap – and batteries. They particularly liked the batteries, because a good number of them were fascinated by torches. Then, when I shut up the shop, they would walk away with me, holding my hand. And at the 'socials', they'd be waiting outside, dying to get in and, when the music started, they'd dance and dance – completely uninhibited. It didn't matter whether they were dancing with someone – they were just happy in themselves. I think that working there taught me an awful lot. You don't have to worry and fret about everything in this life."

From The Second World War Until The Early 1980s

The Social Club

Robin Ballard has provided more information about another development at Princess Christian – the Hospital's Social Club. "The Hospital was always aiming to add things for the patients to do. In the 1970s a Social Club was established which operated principally from the Pitman Hall. A suspended ceiling had been added around the late 1950s – not least to make the heating a little more effective. It had previously looked like an old barn with all the roof timbers visible. Weekly film shows took place on a Tuesday evening, available for any of the residents who wished to attend. The films were hired each week and shown using two projectors to avoid a break in the film, as at least two reels were supplied for each film. By about 1970, the Social Club was expanded and an extension was added to the Pitman Hall to accommodate a lounge and a bar plus a snooker room and other facilities." One local lady, a member of the League of Friends, remembers the residents performing a play there and, over the years, the Local Amateur Dramatic Society (LAMPS) came to do various performances. Joy Dolling recalls that, when she was a teenager, she was part of a cabaret. "At the end, we did three dances as the finale – including the Charleston and the Can-Can. We had very short skirts and the usual frilly knickers. When we finished with the splits, the 'boys' went mad – I don't think that they got much of that type of thing – all the helpers had to calm them down. But it was fun." Pat and Anne Davies had lived initially at Meadway in Hildenborough before moving virtually next door to Princess Christian in Riding Lane.

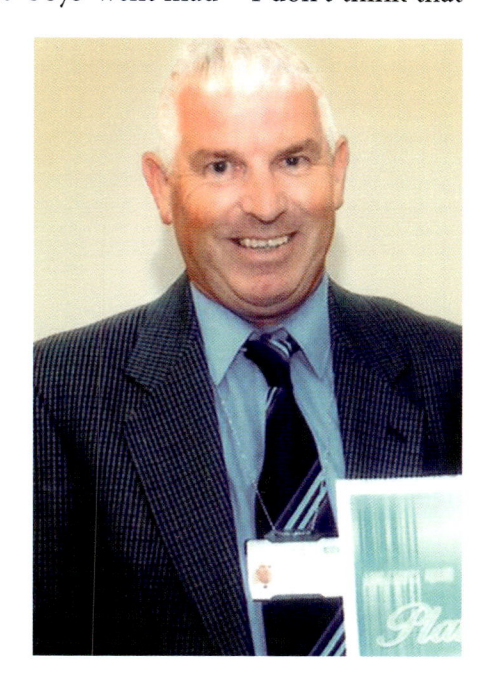

Robin Ballard receiving Long Service Award c.2005. He retired after 34 years working in the NHS.

They have further memories of the social life at Princess Christian. When they first arrived in the area, their neighbour was Ursula Taylor, a Staff Nurse at Princess Christian and they were soon invited to an Open Day. "We were quite nervous when we arrived and were surrounded as we parked the car. When we got out we were hugged and led to the Hall by the residents – who, of course, were only being friendly. It took a bit of getting used to but later when we moved to Riding Lane, we became good friends with all these same people." Pat adds that for several years, he worked in the Bar on New Year's Eve. "Residents could buy their own drinks – they got their own pocket money – and staff were there too. It was all very cheerful. There was one man who went round the ashtrays and collected the dog ends which he made into cigarettes using his roller machine that you used to see in those days. And I remember an old lady who conned me. She ordered a drink but when I told her the price, she scarpered – with the drink – and an evil little laugh. I also noticed a strange, short, round nursing assistant lady. She ended up causing the biggest scandal ever. Her husband was a slim, gentle, fair-haired chap who used to help behind the Bar. But one day he was found murdered and dumped at the Shipbourne end of the Hildenborough Road. The wife was eventually convicted of arranging – and assisting in – his murder with the help of her two teenage lodgers."

In the late 1970s and early 1980s the Social Club was expanded still further. The main area of the Pitman Hall was now large enough for a whole range of activities, both educational and recreational to take place. There were reading classes and speech therapy; and an expanded library. In the good sized kitchen there were regular cooking classes organized by outside volunteers. Mr Cooper was proud of these new developments. For a short time, too, the Social Club acted as an emergency dormitory and then as a Staff Dining Room – but these were only temporary arrangements.

The League of Friends

A League of Friends had been established for many years. One of its aims was to encourage a wider selection of the outside world to become involved. 'Friends' included members of staff, residents' relatives, local people and some student groups such as the VSU (Voluntary Service Units) from Tonbridge School and from several schools and voluntary groups in Sevenoaks, who were interested in the Hospital and helping the community. A second objective of the Friends was to raise funds to help pay for outings and entertainment not covered by NHS funding; and sometimes funding for 'extras' in residents' rooms. The third objective – together with the Social Club – was to organize the many events, both weekly social gatherings and the special outings.

The names of the people we know about who organized the League of Friends, nearly all locals, deserve a mention. It is clear from the few in-house journals that remain that the group had its ups and downs with regard to the number of volunteers it could muster for the actual Committee but it usually seemed to attract a good number of local people to its various dances or balls; its Guy Fawkes bonfire night; its summer barbecues; and the fêtes and Christmas Parties that it arranged. Leading the Committee for twenty or thirty years as its Chairman was Tony Langdon-Down, a solicitor who lived locally and who was the son of Dr Reginald and grandson of Dr John. Even when he retired in 1982 to make way for the energetic Sid Adams, Tony continued as Patron until Princess Christian's closure. Mr G Horsfield, Mrs Mollie Buss and Mr J Hulett did their stints as Hon Sec and Miss G. Parry Morgan as Hon Treasurer in the 1980s. Mrs Jill Scott, later to found the Scott's Project, a centre in Tonbridge for people with learning disabilities, was a member of the League of Friends and for many years in the 1970s and 1980s Mrs Hume, who lived in Mill Lane, was a tireless fighter for the League and for improvements at Princess Christian. Additionally, Mrs Vidler is thanked in a newsletter for giving £500 which mainly was spent on some new swings. The Butt family were also clearly involved. But there must have been many others who were involved to whom history can only thank in a general way.

To give some specific examples of the work of the League of Friends: the autumn 1978 edition of the quarterly house magazine 'Spotlight' gives the League of Friends' income as £850, much of which came from the Summer Open Day, although another major source of revenue for a number of years around the 1960s was a public dance organized by the League of Friends at The Old Barn in Hildenborough, a well-known local venue, capable of holding over two hundred people. The 'Spotlight' article shows the wide range of the extra things that the Friends had been able to provide. There was improved lighting for the Pitman Hall stage, Christmas decorations in the wards and a major firework display. Each resident was given an Easter egg and a Christmas present; and a present and card on his or her birthday, valuable not least because a proportion of the residents did not have any known relatives, or at least none that came to visit or communicate in any way. There was also the maintenance of the colour TVs and – with the Social Club – outings and the film showings. One resident, Bert Wilmore, wrote about that year's June barbecue, "... thank you for the very happy evening we all had at Glen House. There were several tables of eatables – hot-dogs, fried eggs, beef burgers – and lots to drink. It was a warm evening, so it was nice being out in the garden, before all going to the Pitman Hall for a dance Three cheers for the staff and Friends for giving us a good time."

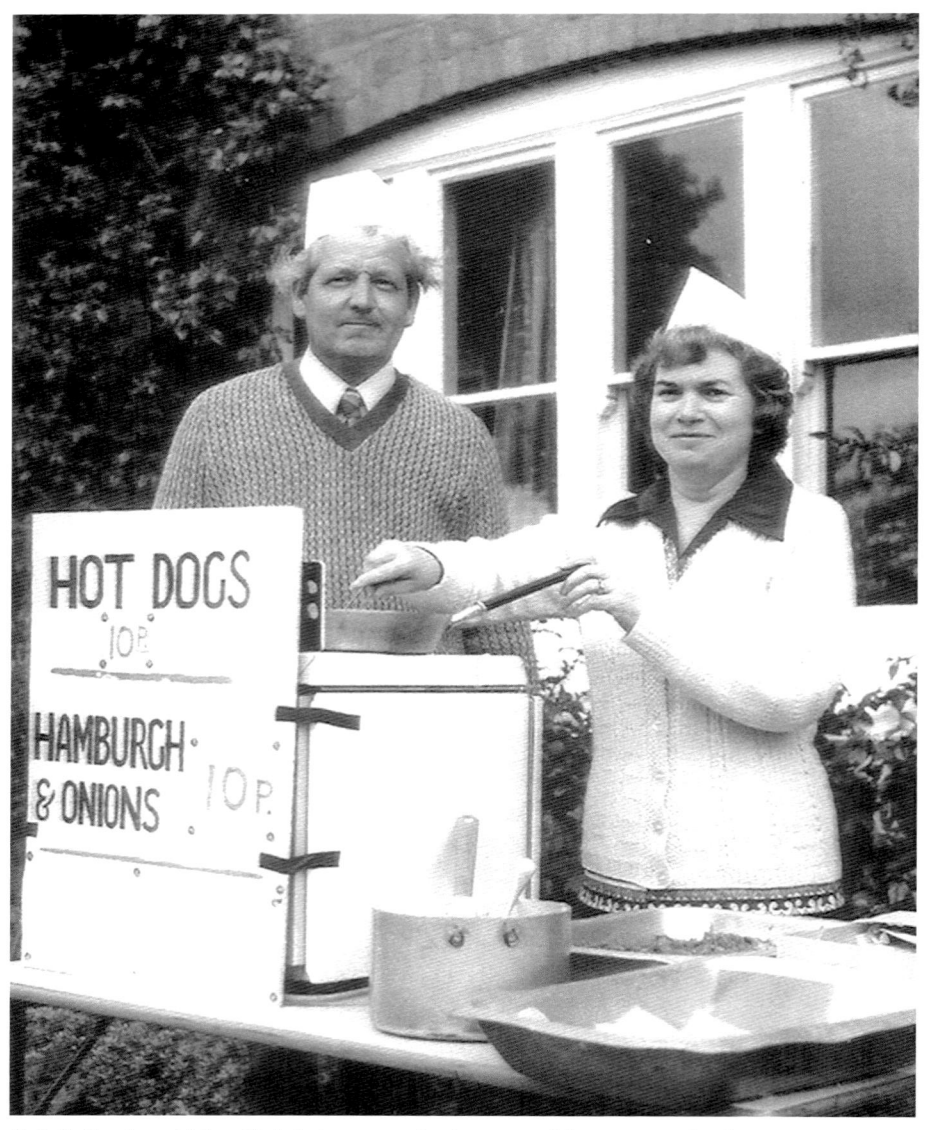

Bob Ballard and his wife helping serve food at one of the summer barbecues.
Photo: Robin Ballard

From The Second World War Until The Early 1980s

THE LEAGUE OF FRIENDS OF PRINCESS CHRISTIAN HOSPITAL
Riding Lane, HILDENBOROUGH, Tonbridge, Kent

(Affiliated to the National League of Hospital Friends)
Registered Charity No 265066

PRESIDENT:	Mr A T Langdon-Down
VICE-PRESIDENT:	Mrs M K E Hume
CHAIRMAN:	Mr Sidney J Adams
HON. TREASURER:	Miss G Parry Morgan, 133 Estridge Way, Tonbridge, Kent
HON. SECRETARY:	Mrs Mollie Buss

ABOUT THE LEAGUE OF FRIENDS

The League is a voluntary organisation which exists to encourage interest in, and service for, the residents, and to support the work of the Hospital staff where possible.

The League provides -

A colour television set for each residential unit and for each resident a birthday card by post and a birthday present delivered personally, an Easter egg and a Christmas present.

It arranges a Fireworks Display and a Christmas Party, and augments refreshments at various events arranged for the residents, i.e. Summer Barbeque.

It has always helped with small and large projects for the benefit and well-being of the residents.

The tightening of public funds will make more calls on the League's resources.

The Financial Year ends on 31 March, and the Annual General Meeting is held in May.

Funds for the League's work are raised mainly from members' subscriptions, donations, social functions, special fund raising activities, and a proportion of the OPEN DAY proceeds. No fixed subscription has been laid down - the Committee feel that this is best left to individual members.

Information on COVENANTS which enable the League to recover the TAX which has been paid by the subscribers can be obtained from the Treasurer.

The formal rules of the League of Friends

In another edition of the house newsletter from 1985, Mollie Buss describes the Bonfire Night Party laid on by the Friends. Residents had been helping collect wood for the bonfire – sited in a safety-conscious place. "On the night, the bonfire is lit and the fireworks, particularly rockets, are set off. There is a kind of magic – perhaps it is in the throng of onlookers – residents and their relatives, Hospital staff at all levels, League of Friends, children, villagers who came in unchallenged, clasping the hands of toddlers muffled to the ears in warm wool? Perhaps it is the large chap next door to you who is assumed to be a resident? He will tell you that the apple trees have been pruned and that those prunings helped to build the huge glowing stack. When the fireworks are over and the fire is dying down just a little beyond the great glow, the evening is not yet over. Residents, and anyone who wishes, may go into the Pitman Hall to the disco where plenty of drinks abound… It is all a time honoured tradition: and sometimes it is important that things do not change…"

The Position in 1981

In 1981 Mr Cooper felt that much had been achieved over the previous ten years. "In 1980/1981 there are 110 males and 48 females who work and play together in all aspects of life here. For years the family atmosphere has been nurtured with both residents and staff. This has not only remained, but has been very much strengthened by this deeply human approach. The visitor will notice the informality and relaxed quality of the regime. It is a truly 'open' community and visitors are always welcome at any time. Many of the residents are able to go out on their own to shop in the village or town or go to football matches, etc, and are well able to look after themselves on buses and are always ready to help other people. The local community accept them in a friendly and neighbourly way. Most people know them and talk quite normally with them. During recent years, the Hospital has organized bigger events in the summer which have brought many hundreds of people inside the grounds, who would have never contemplated this even a few years ago. The results have been encouraging. The residents mix easily with everyone, which has been an 'eye-opener' to many outsiders who have been somewhat apprehensive of coming into this type of community and have shut their eyes to the fact that such places exist."

Some long-term local residents would perhaps have not quite agreed with the last part of this statement but it is true, as Mr Cooper, says that between 1949 and 1981 great strides had been made with involving the community. In reality, for at least forty years most local people had become used to and very often fond of the men and women in Princess Christian. But staff must have felt that the increased policy of openness had indeed persuaded extra outsiders to appreciate the work being done and persuaded a good number of people to join in in an active way. One newsletter said, "In 1980/1981 there has been much building work and structural alternations taking place, and in the near future, the Farm Villa residents will be re-housed in what were the Administration Block and the residents' staff quarters. Thanks to the generosity of a local person, the Oast House Villa now has its own Dining Room, the residents enjoying their first meal in it as lunch on Christmas Eve, 1980. A new dormitory is being built for the residents in the Oast House."

Mr Cooper summarized the position as he saw it in 1981, "All in all, Princess Christian is a busy little hospital where it all seems to be happening, yet still retaining its family atmosphere, peace and tranquillity. Who know what its future prospects are?"

The Princess Christian Hospital Main Site Buildings, 1980 onwards.
Map adapted from Ordnance Survey 4th Edition by John Donald

1. Main Entrance
2. Garages and store rooms
3. North and South Cottages (semi detached)
4. Occupational Therapy huts. Later 'Sensory Room', approx 1990 on.
5. Original farm house – Trench House – which became the Superintendent's house and admin HQ before becoming a men's hostel
6. Shop at one time
7. The Oast House from 1908 – for men
8. Covered passageway
9. New larger bath/washing/toilets for Oast House
10. New dining room for Oast House
11. Bike shed
12. Kitchen (originally laundry)
13. Dining Room
14. Pitman Hall
15. Social Club
16. Offices for senior staff
17. Chicken Houses
18. Glen House (originally the Girls' Home 1917 on)
19. Sewing Room (wooden hut)
20. Pond
21. Hilden Brook
22. Bridge to Glen House
23. Riding Lane to Shipbourne
24. Riding Lane to Farm and Vines Lane; and down to Hildenborough and the main Tonbridge to Sevenoaks road.
25. Public Bridleway
26. Public Footpath

— 114 —

The Princess Christian Main Site and Farm, 1980 onwards.

Map adapted from Ordnance Survey 4th Edition by John Donald

1 Entrance
2 Main Princess Christian buildings
3 Glen House
4 Vines Lane
5 Cottages for 5 men and 5 women (end 1980s)
6 Chestnuts (Staff)
7 Oak Lodge (staff)
8 Three bungalows ('Turnbull Cottages'). Originally staff.
9 Alexander House
10 The Farm and Farm Shop
11 The Hostel/Farm Cottages
12 Barnfield
13 Riding Lane
14 Riding Lane towards Shipbourne
15 Riding Lane to Hildenborough (and Club Cottages and Brownways Cottage)
16 Orchard
17 Hilden Brook

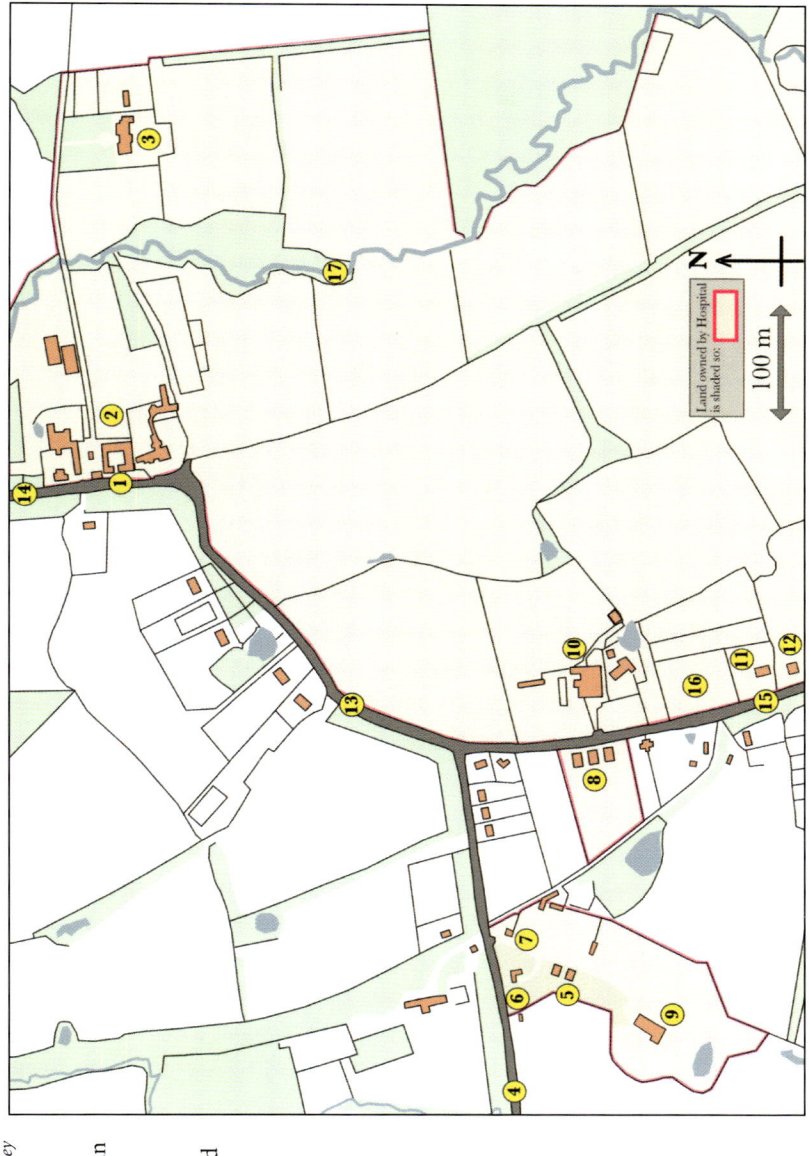

— 115 —

CHAPTER 4
Moving Towards the Closure of Princess Christian: 1981–1995

The Inspector Calls: The 1983 Report

As if to answer Mr Cooper's question – "who knows what the future prospects are?" – an outside team of NHS experts arrived in 1983 and made clear recommendations. There must have been regular inspections of the hospital by outsiders – it was, after all, part of the NHS – but we do not know how often or what they reported. However, the Library of the Maidstone & Tunbridge Wells NHS Trust has found this unpublished Report[75] which puts into context many of the subjects already discussed. It is certainly not flattering about a good number of aspects of the Hospital and its management; but it was the job of the inspectors to safeguard the individuals at the Hospital. So what were the inspectors' main thoughts? On the positive side they started by saying that "the basic physical care being provided was of a good standard…". However, the sentence continues, "but uninspired and traditional nursing attitudes gave the impression that this rural community had been standing still for many years." They go on to express their dismay at the lack of more systematic education and training to help residents progress into the wider world, blaming a combination of poor management structures, lack of money and too few staff, most of whom did not receive proper training. Leybourne Grange is indirectly criticized for not providing enough expertise and leadership. The inspectors felt that this lack of training for the residents was particularly unfortunate as a large proportion of them – probably two thirds – would be able, with better 'education', to be living within the newly proposed 'Community Care' structure. The inspectors did admit that the residents seemed happy and that relatives of the residents thought the Hospital looked after its patients well. The Hildenborough GP practice is praised; and additionally, the inspectors felt that the good work being done at the Farm could be expanded to provide training for day-students from other parts of the area.

There are several tables of statistics. The first shows that there were one hundred and sixty beds of which one hundred and fifty-four were occupied. (No sub-division into men and women is given.) The second table analyzes the age of the residents where 53% were aged sixteen to forty-nine; 34% were between fifty and sixty-four; and 13% were over sixty-five. (One guesses that quite a high proportion of the twenty or so oldest patients had been at Princess Christian for most of their adult lives and there is some later evidence to this effect.) A further table analyzes those with special needs – mainly physical problems such as the inability to walk, incontinence, blindness; and a final table which gives the actual numbers of nursing staff and what is the much higher figure of staff who should be employed.

Perhaps one of the most interesting points in the Report – partly a query and partly a suggestion – arises almost at the end of the document. It raises the question that, as the inspectors were recommending two-thirds of the residents should be resettled in the community, how and where should the remaining third be looked after? This seems to imply that maybe fifty people had to be retained within some sort of small hospital. As we will see, this did not happen. The inspectors assessed the patients individually, placing them in one of four 'Groups' under what was then called the Wessex Scale.[76]

Group I people: are "competent in all areas of self-help; they are ambulant and continent; they have no behaviour problems and are not disruptive in any way. They could be discharged home or to a hostel immediately without any special facilities necessary, apart from those normally provided in a local authority hostel. Some may be appropriately placed in group homes." The inspectors reckoned that fifty-eight (39%) of Princess Christian residents fell within this category.

Group II people: are described as "continent, ambulant and almost completely self-sufficient. They may have mild problems of behaviour but these could be corrected with a short period of treatment and some self-help training ... [These people] should be suitable for immediate discharge home or to a hostel, where, after a short period of pre-discharge training, they would be suitable for discharge to a group home or other forms of independent living in the community." Sixty-five residents (42%) were considered to fall within this classification. So, taking Group I and Group II residents together, there were one hundred and twenty-three people or 81% of Princess Christian's men and women who the inspectors felt did not need to be in the Hospital.

Group III people: are "generally continent but with lapses at night. Some are mildly over-active, with occasional mild behaviour problems. All are said to be easily managed and would benefit from specific training. If discharged to a hostel, the staff ratio would need to be higher than for those in Groups I and II." (Elsewhere in the Report it recommends that Group III staff/resident ratio should be 1:4 as opposed to Groups I and II which are respectively 1:8 and 1:6.) Only twelve residents were classified as Group III.

Group IV people: are classified as "severe double incontinent, with multiple physical handicaps including severe epilepsy, extreme hyperkinetic behaviour and/or aggression to themselves or to others. The majority require some form of long-term residential care with a high staff/resident ratio". (Elsewhere in the Report the ratio is given as 1:1). There were eighteen residents classified as Group IV, although later in the Report, it mentions that only seven had severe behavioural problems, with the other eleven presumably primarily having major physical problems as well as the learning disabilities. The relatively low numbers of people with severe physical problems (Group IV) was likely to be partly explained by the choices made by the experts at Leybourne years earlier, when they had selected people with less severe learning and physical difficulties. Those in Group III and Group IV were probably mainly the more elderly who had been at Princess Christian for many years.

The largest part of the Report reflects concern about the paucity of the training at Princess Christian, which was meant to help residents live a life in the outside world.. A number of reasons for this and recommendations are made including the need for more money and for more staff (whilst commenting that the provision of more staff was unlikely).

One person who very much agreed with the part of the 1983 Report which commented on the lack of preparation for 'Care in the Community' was Ann Trigg (although she never saw the Report). Ann had arrived at Leybourne in 1984 to be in charge of occupational therapy at both Leybourne and Princess Christian. Much of her work was to ensure that as many residents as possible from both hospitals were made ready to live in the wider world. "I was really surprised when I first visited Princess Christian. The attitudes of both the senior people and the care staff felt like the Dark Ages. The staff were all really caring. The atmosphere was peaceful and happy, but there was very little training of the residents to prepare them for the future of 'Care in the Community' which everyone knew was coming. They didn't see the move into the community in a positive light. They saw themselves as caring guardians, rather than helping the residents develop skills they would need for the future. I got to know a good number of the residents and I remember talking with an elderly lady. She regularly read the newspapers and was very clear-headed. She had been there for years and once I asked her how she had first come to be at Princess Christian. She told me that her mother had died when she was seventeen and that her father hadn't been able to cope. So she got sent to Princess Christian. Another had stolen a packet of cigarettes. But for such people, who had been looked after totally by the staff for a great many years, it was not going to be easy to get them trained to be able to look after themselves – even if the staff had thought about it. The trouble was that the authorities had not trained the staff to look at things for the future. I remember I started to prepare for cooking lessons and some of the staff were horrified. 'You can't do that', they said and I asked 'why not?' and one of them said, 'You don't know where their hands have been.' And I said, 'Well, I don't know where your hands have been and anyway that's the first thing I'll be teaching them – wash your hands before you start cooking.' But we did get progress and as the winding down of Princess Christian continued, Carolyn Schwitzer, the new full-time OT person who arrived in 1989 at Princess Christian was a great help. We used to select a group of two or four residents who came from the same area and get them ready to move into the outside world together. With luck they still had relatives or people they knew near where they were going to live but at least they'd have each other. So in the end, it worked out, although the changeover was not always easy. But today the system seems to be working well in nearly all cases. (Incidentally, you mentioned all the different words for people with not very serious learning disabilities. Have you been told about 'dongers' or 'dungers' – I don't know how you should spell it. It was a Leybourne term for the less able who wore dungarees as a uniform.)"

In common with other aspects of the Hospital, by the late 1970s and early 1980s the state of some of the facilities and buildings was less than ideal. Much was not up to the standard expected of an NHS hospital. The 1983 Report had drawn attention to the fact that "the general fabric of the buildings was poor due to little capital development… a lack of manpower… and the Sevenoaks sector, which [should have provided the money], left an inadequate share for Princess Christian." And indeed, the position was to get worse. As the 1980s progressed and residents began to be moved out, the active policy of neglect for buildings and facilities which were, or were soon to be, redundant, continued – perhaps not unnaturally but clearly it was less than ideal for the remaining staff and residents.

The Transfer of the Farm from the NHS to Kent County Council

Whilst the plans to implement 'Care in the Community' and to close down what were called mental institutions – in this case Leybourne and Princes Christian – were taking shape, the NHS became concerned that, as a medical organization, they should not really be running a farm. The Report by the outside experts had praised the Farm and the work that it did. It had said that a number of Princess Christian's residents had been so successfully trained at the Farm that they had been able to move to outside jobs, including work on normal farms. The Report mentioned that there were currently fifty-five cattle, a developing beef herd, thirty-five calves, sixty-six weaner piglets for fattening and a thousand poultry with a hundred and ten acres for hay. Residents were still being introduced to farming work by taking responsibility for either a new-born calf or a group of weaner piglets; and they learnt about feeding, cleaning and rearing the animals. They then had the opportunity to specialize in pigs, poultry or dairy work. The organization came under the Manager, John Clayton, who was assisted by a full-time tractor driver, a cowman and lady who specialized in the pig and poultry side. However, the Report went on to point out that, out of the hundred and sixty residents at Princess Christian, only thirty-four – thirty-two men and two women – worked on the Farm and the number seemed likely to decrease. It was noted that there were increasing numbers of people from the outside who came to work on a daily basis, referred to the Farm by social services; and the inspectors thought that this trend would and should increase. They formally recommended that the Farm be transferred to social services. All the pieces of the jigsaw were, therefore, coming together and, after lengthy debate, Kent County Council Social Services agreed to take over the Farm. At the beginning of October 1987, the Kent and Sussex Courier reported that the Chairman of Tunbridge Wells Health Authority, Sir John Grugeon, formally handed over the Farm with twenty-five acres to Mr Bill McNeill, the Chairman of the Kent County Council. At this time the article reported that the Farm was producing fruit, vegetables and flowers, as well as rearing the poultry, pigs and calves – and rabbits. There were also classes in domestic science for men and woman.[77]

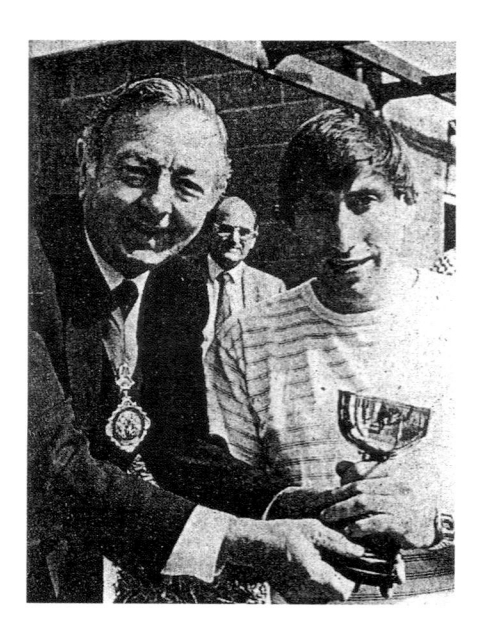

Caption: The Chairman of Kent County Council, Mr Bill McNeill, presents the Endeavour Cup to Princess Christian Farm Trainee Colin Cox during the farm's transfer to the county council on Friday
Photo: Kent and Sussex Courier, 2 October 1987.

However, the original land purchased in the 1904-1910 period[78] comprised of over 120 acres. With the 1987 transfer of the Farm with its twenty-five acres to Social Services, it was agreed that the remaining ninety-five acres would be let out by the NHS to local farmers – not least because this land had become very run down. No maintenance had been carried out for a number of years. The hedges were overgrown; weeds had taken over the pasture; fences and gates were broken or badly rusted away; and trees blown down in the 1987 storm littered fields. Unfortunately, over the next few years the state of this land was found to be so poor that the local farmers found it uneconomic to use it and the last farmer with grazing rights gave it up in 1990. So, in a new agreement between the Kent County Council and the NHS, the land was taken back and in 1991 the Farm was allowed to use it at a rent of £2,281 a year for grazing rights. However, once again the state of the land was found to be in poorer condition than first thought. So in 1992 it was agreed that the Farm could have the land rent-free for the next three years on condition that the Farm re-did the hedges and fencing and improved the quality of the pasture. At the end of three years, the rent would be renegotiated depending on progress achieved. It was also agreed that the farm would start a nature trail over the land which could be used by people with learning disabilities and people in wheelchairs. In due course, this trail was built with help from some of the residents at Princess Christian and the improvements which had been discussed were completed.

Moving Towards the Closure of Princess Christian: 1981–1995

In spite of these changes in the organization of the Farm, the 'boys' and, occasionally, the 'girls', continued the work that they loved on the Farm. In 1987, a News In Focus article gave a good example of what was actually happening now that the Farm was being run by the Kent County Council.[79] The article describes the wide range of work on the Farm and also to explain that the farm hands nowadays came not only from the Hospital but also from local hostels for people who needed extra help and experience to obtain a job. The policy recommended in the 1983 Inspectors' Report was being implemented. The article goes on to describe "how vegetables are grown, sometimes in polytunnels, how chickens are raised for their eggs and how the pigs, calves and rabbits are reared, with all the produce sold to local Kent County Council establishments as well as to pubs and restaurants in the area." The photographs accompanying the article give a good feeling of the men and the work, and the pride that the workers on the Farm felt.

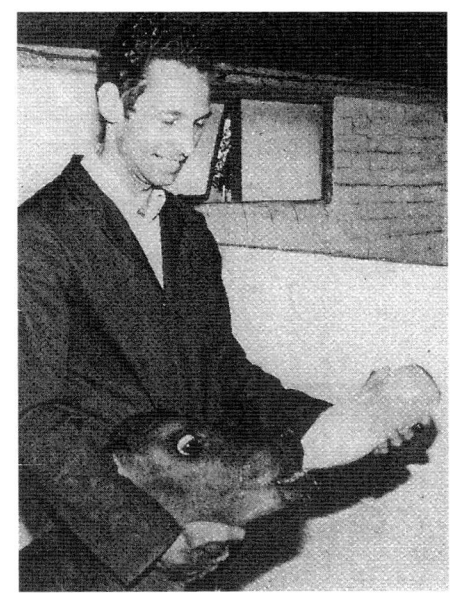

A calf gets to grips with bottle feeding helped by Tommy Newson.

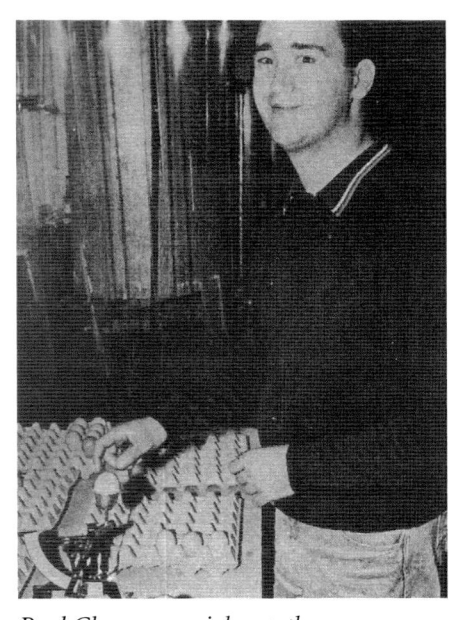

Paul Channon weighs up the eggs grading situation.

Photos: from Kent and Sussex Courier 29 – 30 September 1987 (pictures by Irene Nicholls)

The farm hands were also working on building new pig sties and were being taught wider living skills. There was a new kitchen where people could learn to cook and there was even a modern video player where a range of subjects could be learnt.

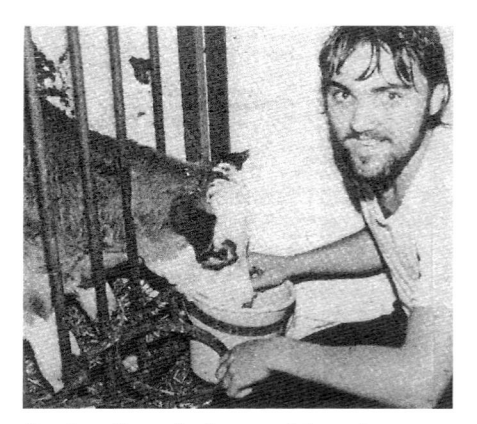

Stephen Pratt feeds one of the calves at the farm.

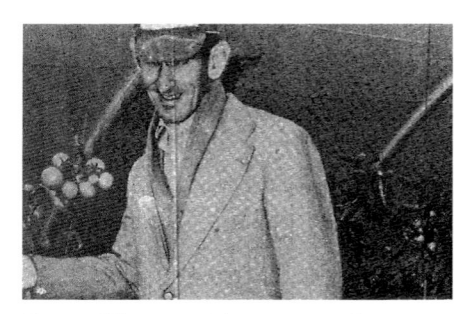

Danny Thomas picks tomatoes from one of the plastic tunnels.

Photos: from Kent and Sussex Courier
29 – 30 September 1987
(pictures by Irene Nicholls)

John Clayton, the Farm Manager, was interviewed: "At Princess Christian we give them a chance to learn skills needed to live in today's society, like cooking and road safety and how to use money. They are taught a variety of farming methods which could help them find agricultural work. The people here enjoy learning and working in our farm environment. It gives them a sense of achievement and enjoyment when they see their plants grow and are given the opportunity to look after animals. Here they have the space or 'elbow room' to live." Another indication of the Farm's success came in December 1988 when the Farm entered the Sevenoaks Fatstock and Sale Show. It took the top award for its pen of three porkers, beating entries from farms as far afield as Essex and Suffolk as well as Kent. At this stage, the 'students' or 'trainees', as they were now called, were raising three hundred piglets a year, many hundreds of chickens, rearing calves and raising a wide variety of plants in the greenhouses.[80] Three years later in the early 1990s the Farm, now with its original acreage restored, was able to expand and to keep up to two hundred sheep – including some hand reared from a week old by bottle – which the residents loved doing; and sixty acres was usually put aside for hay which was sold in the winter to riding stables and other outlets as well as being used on the Farm itself. The Farm Shop, which had been started on a very small scale some years earlier, was expanded – including selling some of the recently cut logs. The Farm was now virtually a separate entity from the Hospital.

The Staff

It would be tidy and useful to be able to record more about the staff, particularly from 1948 to the early 1990s: but, as so often in this book, there are no formal documents and only a few issues of the in-house magazines, together with the memories from some of the people who worked at Princess Christian. An Appendix gives a very incomplete list of the staff where I have been given them and it would be useful for further editions to have more names. So more details, please. It would also be helpful to know more about the staff structure and the ratio of staff to the residents. The staffing seems to have been divided into two types of people – the main care staff together with the cooks, domestic and admin staff – and outsiders – including the qualified medical nurses on duty call over the twenty-four hours a day, who in practical terms came under the outside GP, who visited several times a week. There were other outsiders, often ladies who helped with practical lessons such as sewing and art. There were visiting experts – physiotherapists and occupational therapists at various periods. There was also a driver. A well-remembered one was Sam, who again was part of the team for a long period.

There has been one – and only one – distressing story about Princess Christian staff. It comes from a very reliable source, and perhaps applied only to an isolated period. A local lady volunteered to help with arts and crafts, working with the new Occupational Therapist. The volunteer was told that there was a regular pre-meeting to decide what was going to be done that day. When she attended the first meeting, she met the relatively new Occupational Therapist, together with four ladies from the care staff who looked after the particular 'girls' who would be coming. However, nothing about the coming day's work was discussed then or ever seemed to be discussed, with the staff sitting around drinking tea and smoking and making derisory remarks about the 'girls'. Meanwhile, the 'girls' themselves were kept waiting outside "even if it was raining or, once, snowing." When the 'girls' were finally allowed in, the staff continued to make hurtful remarks about them to their faces. The lady volunteer stuck this for several months and then left. The Occupational Therapist left soon after. These comments are verified by the lady volunteer's husband. Both were long-term supporters of the Colony. Over the past few years there have been reports in the national news about ill treatment by staff in either old people's care homes or of patients in long-stay hospitals. For any visitor who has spent time in a care home or an old people's home, the staff have virtually all seemed caring, whatever the seemingly overwhelming problems with individual patients.

The Princess Christian Farm Colony and Hospital 1895–1995

Yet clearly there are a very small proportion of staff, who for some difficult to explain reason, have abandoned decency. It is sad to find this could have occurred at Princess Christian at one point in time – particularly when every other report has said how totally caring and committed the staff were.

One of the most moving accounts of the day-to-day working at Princess Christian comes from Hildenborough's most famous son – in this case, daughter – Kelly Holmes. It is taken from her extremely readable autobiography, "Black, White and Gold"[81] and relates to her time after leaving school and before going into the Army in 1987, a time when Princess Christian was just starting to wind down. However, as is clear from this account, the residents were still being looked after with the greatest care. The extract is reproduced with Kelly's permission.

"I started working at the Princess Christian hospital for mentally handicapped adults when I was seventeen. Mum worked nights there as an auxiliary nurse but during the day I was a nursing assistant. There were various wards that each dealt with different levels of problems with both men and women. I worked with Nan Connor, who was head of the department, and Deirdre Morgan, an auxiliary nurse, at one of the hospital buildings called the Oast House in which the patients were all men aged anything from twenty to seventy years old. One of my jobs was to help them into the shower, wash them, help them out, dry them and dress them. I had to teach them about using toilet paper as well as washing their hands. The Oast House had a very long lounge with two round turrets at either end. The men would all sit on their chairs in there except for Eric who paced up and down with a big smile on his face, holding his ears and making a 'brrr' noise. At the end was the small office where Nan worked, organising the ward, ordering meals and making sure all hospital appointments were kept. To the left was a large bathroom area that contained toilet cubicles, a shower and a big bath, with a chair-lift and cupboards for all the patients' clothes, which we neatly folded and stacked, carefully labelling them with name tags for each patient.

"There were around twenty men, all of different abilities and personalities. Two of the patients particularly touched my heart. One was a smoker who used to get taken down to the newsagents to buy his cigarettes. I spent a lot of time chatting with him and decided I would teach him about money, which he didn't understand at all. We practised and practised until he knew exactly how much he needed for the cigarettes and for the bus fare to the newsagents and back. At last D-day arrived, I took him to the bus stop outside the hospital and waited for the bus with him. Then off he went on his own. I had already called the newsagents to warn them he was coming and to ask them to be sure that he was given the right brand of cigarettes and the right change, and that he got on the right bus back. While he was gone, I waited nervously inside the main hospital building where I could see the bus stop. At last the bus came into view and pulled up outside. The doors swished open and out he stepped, proud as punch at having managed the journey all on his own. It was fantastic to have helped him achieve this new level of independence. I never knew whether he was able to keep doing it after I left but at least he had done it once and knew that he could. The other man, Johnny Bray, was a lively Down's syndrome guy in his late sixties. Over the time he'd been in the hospital, he had physically deteriorated and, by the time I knew him, he was hunched over in a wheelchair. When he was moved to our ward, I used to take him to Rehab where he'd be strapped on to a bench that was tipped upright to straighten him up. After a couple of hours of standing like this, he was able to walk a few steps. I used to volunteer to go with him whenever I could. I'd spend the time playing games and puzzles with him on the tray that was set up in front of him. Then, when his time was up, the staff would release him and he'd walk towards me with a huge beaming smile on his face. It was so brilliant to see him doing this that I'd have tears rolling down my cheeks. I'd seen photos of him dancing around and it seemed so unfair that although he still seemed full of life, he could do so little. Three weeks after I'd left to join the Army, one of the staff phoned me to tell me that Johnny had died. I was heartbroken. But I've never forgotten him. Helping these men towards little improvements in their lives was one of the most rewarding jobs I've ever had. It was also a demanding job, and it made me appreciate how hard doctors and nurses in hospitals must work."

Kelly Holmes' account and other accounts in this book may make it sound as if there were a good number of staff to look after the patients. However, in reality there were surprisingly few carers, bearing in mind the number of residents, the variety of accommodation buildings and the need for twenty-four hour oversight, let alone the need for training to help the 'boys' and 'girls' go out in the community. In the 1983 Report,[82] the outside experts gave their views about the number and type of nursing staff needed to cope properly with the one hundred and fifty-three residents. It contrasted these figures with the actual number employed. In essence, it says that around seventy-three nursing staff should be employed. Instead, there were fifty-four actually in post. So Princess Christian was dramatically understaffed in respect of nurses. Because the Report contains one of the few pieces of factual information about the Princess Christian staffing levels, the section is given in full on the following page:

At the time of our visit, nursing services at Princess Christian's were being restructured. It was proposed that there should be three nursing officers for Princess Christian's, one with manager responsibility for day duty, one for night duty, and the other in charge of resident training. We recommend that one nursing officer should assume overall responsibility for the nursing service at Princess Christian's and should be responsible to the Director of Nursing Services. At the time of our visit the total nursing establishment was 53.99 WTEs,[83] 36.5% of whom were trained nurses. The following table gives the recommended establishment for Princess Christian's based on an analysis of dependency of the residents:

Recommended Nursing Establishment

	No of Residents	Staff/Resident Ratio	Recommended Establishment (WTE)
Group I	58	1:8	7
Group II	65	1:6	11
Group III	12	1:4	3
Group IV	18	1:1	18
Sub-Total			**39**
Plus 26% for sickness, training, leave, etc			10
Plus night duty (current establishment)			16.5
Plus training areas (current establishment)			8
Total Recommended Establishment			**73.5 WTE**[84]

The shortfall of nursing staff between our recommended establishment based on resident dependency and the funded establishment was 19.61. We appreciate that the funding to increase the establishment of nursing staff will be almost impossible to find. Nevertheless there is a clear indication of how the present staff are stretched. A mini manpower study using our analysis of dependency should be carried out to ensure that existing staff are deployed as effectively as possible.

Moving Towards the Closure of Princess Christian: 1981–1995

The above assessment is primarily concerned with what was thought to be an inadequate level of staff who did the actual nursing. However, in another part of the Report it states that "support services to help the nursing staff were badly lacking and in particular domestic services were not available…". Added to the Report's conclusion that maintenance and works staff were overstretched, it is clear Princess Christian did not have enough people to do as complete a job as the Report was recommending or the Hospital's management would have liked.

There is only one further mention of staffing levels post World War II in the papers which do exist and it reflects the views of an insider. It comes in a cheerful piece about events over the past year, 1982, and was written by a staff member who appears to be relatively senior – Charles Billington. (In the several articles we have from him, he comes across as a whimsical and cheerful man, totally dedicated to the Princess Christian community). In this particular article he describes the holidays taken by residents "at Hastings, Isle of Sheppey, Broadstairs, etc – resorts which are relatively near. Although some of these holidays may sound old fashioned, we have a party of twenty or so residents with four or five staff." He contrasts these ratios of residents to staff while away on a holiday with the ratio at Princess Christian which he says was normally much less. He goes on to look at the future, suggesting that, in these difficult and changing times (1982), "there seems to be emerging, amidst the possible gloom of confusion, one positive ideal behind which many of us could come together. Surely we should find some responsible means to campaign for a BETTER ratio of staff to residents in the new era to which we progress? Surely to do otherwise would be to continue a form of cruelty and deprivation to our residents." This thought, from a cheerful and constructive man, does remind us of the strains that staff must have often been under.

Yet there is another way of looking at staff. The ratio of staff to residents may have been too small, the hours of work long and pay almost certainly low, (although not one person has mentioned their wages). However, it seems that the staff loved their jobs and many of them stayed for many years. In another 1984 in-house magazine which covered both Princess Christian and Leybourne Grange, there is a short item headed 'With Regret'. A man had just died who had been a driver at Leybourne from 1934 to 1965. Another man had been a gardener from 1936 to 1975. And a third had been a charge nurse from 1937 until 1978. All had regularly returned in their retirement to visit not only their old friends amongst the staff but old friends amongst the residents – some of whom they must have known well for thirty or forty years. But, however little we know about these people, society owes the Princess Christian staff a considerable debt for their commitment.

'Care in the Community' Explained

Although the general policy of moving towards the winding down of all asylums and mental institutions had been accepted since the 1970s, it was only in the early/mid 1980s that the effects began to be seen at Princess Christian. The detailed explanation of the new policy for West Kent was described by W. (Bill) Cowell, the Director of Nursing Services at Leybourne and, indirectly, in charge of Princess Christian, in an article in the autumn 1984 issue of the quarterly newsletter, Spotlight (see Appendix 4). It is clear from other documents that many staff were perturbed. They had spent ten or often twenty years or more looking after the patients at Princess Christian, trying with great dedication to help each individual there on a personal basis. Staff clearly realized that the new plans – however admirable in theory – were going to change not only their own lives but the lives of the hundred and fifty patients most of whom regarded Princess Christian as the only home they had ever known. Against this background, Mr Cowell realized that he had to try to reassure staff, as well as inform them. He starts by saying that nothing is totally clear-cut as yet and staff views are welcome. He then goes on to tell staff about how the national policy will be translated into action so that, over a ten year period, patients at Leybourne Grange and Princess Christian will be moved into small units, either private care homes or Social Services residential units. The aim will be to keep patients near to relatives or where their roots are. To close both hospitals will mean re-housing around seventy patients from the two hospitals each year. "Some disruption and change to the lives of both residents and staff is inevitable," although in total more staff would be needed under the new arrangements; and there will be staff re-training. He concludes by praising staff for their dedication in the past but making it clear that community care – while in its infancy – is the right way forward. Perhaps the only point that he does not make is the fact that over the previous twenty or thirty years, new medical treatments, particularly new drugs, had made it very much easier for patients with learning disabilities to live a relatively normal life within the community.

It is difficult to know how Mr Cowell's relatively well-reasoned plan was received by staff. Perhaps separate letters should have been sent to the staff at Leybourne and at Princess Christian. Perhaps they were. However, change and managing change, as has often been said, is never straightforward. Formal access to the various committee papers which guided the new plans over the next years is not possible but a small, random selection – clearly from individuals who had received them – is lodged in the Kent Archives and recipients of the papers have written comments in the margins – usually dubious. "How?" is a fairly typical query from people who were going to be implementing the various committee edicts. What is clear, however, is that the individuals on the ground, as well as the management, who would have to provide sensitive and practical care to guide Leybourne and Princess Christian over the coming ten years, had a huge task.

Bill Cowell had been in charge at Leybourne Grange for many years. By coincidence, he lived in Hildenborough, and his wife did occasional nursing at Princess Christian. One community nurse, who had a good deal to do with Leybourne, describes him as greatly liked and respected. She said that he knew the names of all the one and a half thousand Leybourne 'residents' and staff and the villas in which the 'residents' lived. In spite of the business-like tone of his letter to the staff of the two hospitals, it would have probably needed a different skill to change from running the two institutions to actually winding them down. The community nurse said that the Trustees/Board brought in a new chief executive – he was ex-Sainsburys – and Bill Cowell moved on to help found the Maidstone Community Mental Handicap team which later became mcch, the organization which has been one of the main charities to provide housing and care of various kinds on behalf of the Kent County Council for the people from Leybourne and Princess Christian as they moved into the community. Here was yet another person who devoted most of his life to helping those with mental health and learning disability problems.

How Change Was Implemented from Winter 1984/85

So it was now up to the authorities to put in place mechanisms, people and money to implement what was going to be a massive change for residents – and a massive change, too, for staff. It is lucky from an historical point of view that we have two articles which describe how the changes were introduced and even some of the names of the people concerned. There are also the first-hand memories of the person who six years later became the Chairman of the Trust that continued the job of winding down Princess Christian in its final stages. (Sadly, there is little from the residents of Princess Christian themselves. In spite of discussing the issue with a number of people, it has not been thought practical or sensitive to talk very much with former resident about their lives twenty-five or thirty years ago.)

The first article appeared in Spotlight, the regular newsletter for staff at the two hospitals. It was written by David Grant and was published six months after Mr Cowell's overall policy statement. David Grant's title at the KCC was Principal Social Worker and he headed a group, established in November 1984, called the Social Work Team. It consisted of six full-time staff and two part-time staff; and its remit sounds enormous. "We are responsible for providing a social work service to mentally handicapped people and their families at Leybourne Grange and Princess Christian and the community in Tonbridge." As this involved over one and a half thousand 'residents' and their families at the two Hospitals and their dispersal into the community AND it seems to have included a range of other social care activities, it is lucky he sounded a forceful character if he was to tackle this enormous task with such a small staff. He goes on. "We are predominantly involved in the rehabilitation of residents, from the two hospitals into the community but our work ranges from dealing with family crises involving a mentally handicapped person, providing a range of practical support services such as short and long-term care in residential homes, places at our Social Education Centres, help with DHSS benefits and other welfare rights issues etc." With this range of work, it is perhaps not surprising that over the coming years, Kent County Council was one of the first social service departments to use the private, charitable sector – closely supervised – to run a number of its mental handicapped or learning disability services. David Grant continues to explain. "Once the residents are discharged into the community, most become the responsibility of the KCC's Social Services Departments, so it seems sensible that the same departments should be involved from the beginning to ensure that any placement made is the right one." While this arrangement seems logical, it must be remembered that the residents at Princess Christian and Leybourne were in NHS hospitals and the change of organization to KCC Social Services Departments involved an extra layer of potential complexity.

How was this all going to be done in practice? David Grant explains, tactfully, again in the regular Leybourne and Princess Christian newsletter. "We rely heavily on the support of nursing staff to help us get to know residents and we actively encourage their participation in the process by taking them to visit placements with the resident. We lay great stress on the fact that the resident, wherever possible and able, should be helped to understand what is going on and to ensure that their views are taken into account." Once again, these aspirations were admirable but one can imagine a middle-aged Down's man or woman who had lived at Princess Christian for many years and who probably had no relatives, being less than keen to go to new sheltered accommodation in an area they did not really know, without the friends and the staff they had lived with, sometimes for the whole of his or her adult life. For example, the year before David Grant's explanations, Joyce Dobell, who had been born in 1918 and who had arrived at Princess Christian aged fifteen in 1933, died aged seventy-five in 1983, still at Princess Christian after fifty years. Would she have welcomed the consultation, let alone the move?

David Grant, not unaware of the challenges he and his team (and the system) faced, goes on to discuss the families. "The same [consultation] applies to the residents' families, as the news that their son or daughter may leave hospital often comes as a shock. It is our job to carefully explain the reasons for this and to offer support and counselling. Most families eventually see that a move for their mentally handicapped relative is desirable and they are supportive of the idea. If we encounter opposition to a move from a resident or their family, then we would not normally discharge the resident. Many people need time to get used to the idea and talking again about the subject a few months later can often make the difference. Community services for people with a mental handicap are gradually developing but are not as 'visible' as the long-stay hospitals. This often causes families some consternation." He was right to mention the anxieties of parents who had children born with learning difficulties. The author has talked with a good number of these parents. It is clear that as well as the short-term practical difficulties that many of them face every single day, including trying to find outside help and the best school for their much loved child, always at the back of their minds is what will happen to the child when they, the parents, grow old and one day die. How will their child, by then an adult, be looked after? The old, long-stay hospitals, with experienced staff and other residents with not dissimilar difficulties around them as their friends, had always seemed the best way forward. David Grant clearly felt there were better alternatives and, in a follow-up book, "Couldn't You Just Call Me John?", which looks thirty years forward to the present day, we will see whether it has been possible to achieve what the social workers sought to do – and still seek to do.

Yet another hurdle in the practical difficulties David Grant and his team faced was the geographical origin of the residents of Princess Christian (and Leybourne). Neither Hospital had been established to take just West Kent people but one of the main objectives of 'Care in the Community' was to have the Hospital residents in their 'own community'. David Grant accepted that the residents in the two Hospitals came not only from Kent but from twenty-one other Local Authorities. "Therefore, the need to make contact with families involves us in extensive travelling…" This problem was even worse when there was no family to visit as we will see in one Princess Christian example later. Additionally, David Grant hints politely that perhaps not all other Local Authorities were up-to-speed with the new developments, although the Government's new Regional Funding Policy had commenced a year earlier in April 1983. He sees it as a vital part of his role to act as "a watchdog with regard to the quality of the placements." After the first year his team already had records of over a hundred placements which they kept up-to-date, although he admitted that these were mainly about higher ability residents. He does not directly mention that there were a further fourteen hundred people to place – but it must have been in his mind. His final plea to his readers – who would have been mainly staff and families at the two Hospitals – was for understanding and help. "Our involvement is sometimes seen as an intrusion and threat to staff who may have been working with the particular resident for years… All the Social Work Team are qualified and experienced in working with mentally handicapped people… We are only few in number but are always happy to spend some time in explaining our work."

The Start of the Main Close Down: 1985 on

However, the new national policy puzzled many local residents. Bill Richardson and Ron Wood, who had both lived in Hildenborough all their lives and had known the 'boys' and 'girls' at Princess Christian for over fifty years are still dubious about the way Princess Christian was wound down – certainly in its initial stages. Both accept that in principle some of the 'colonists' could have lived fairly normal lives under the proposed 'Care in the Community' system but both agreed with the widely held view that the 'colonists' were very happy at Princess Christian. "It was their home; and for most of them, it was all they knew," says Ron. Bill adds, "It was not a good idea – it was cruel – to send some of them off to places where they didn't know anyone."

In the later 1970s and throughout the 1980s, Princess Christian and Leybourne Grange sought the involvement of teenagers, either through individual schools or through Voluntary Service Units, who would visit the

Moving Towards the Closure of Princess Christian: 1981–1995

Hospitals on a regular basis. The idea was not so much that the teenagers undertook 'work' – much more that they learnt to be more understanding about mentally handicapped people and were able to provide friendship to residents perhaps for a year or even two. It was informal and included the dances and outings as well as chatting to individuals. In the first half of the 1980s, two sisters from Leigh were part of the Sevenoaks Voluntary Service Unit that used to visit Princess Christian every Friday or Sunday, as well as going to social events and helping to organize the various trips. They chatted with the patients and got to know them as individuals. They also used to go over to Leybourne on a regular basis. One of the sisters recalls – with pleasure – what they used to do. "I remember there was one enormous man – I think he was called George – and, directly we got there, he would rush up and hug us. He was so strong he'd almost crush the breath out of us. And there was a lady who was always, always knitting. She never seemed to stop. We got very fond of our own 'little old men'. We also went to Leybourne Grange but that could be grimmer. Once or twice we saw the wards where some of them lived. There were some patients who were confined to their cots. It was rather distressing but I suppose they had to be there and looked after in that way." The younger Leigh sister continues. "But what really upset both me and my sister was when we were told all of a sudden that the Hospital – the Home – was going to be shut down and the people we had grown fond of were just going to be sent away. We asked about it and were told that there was a new policy to put Down's syndrome people in small residential houses – four or six of them with a sort of matron or with carers, depending on how capable they were of looking after themselves. We were so upset that Princess Christian was going to be wound down and I was particularly upset to find that my special old man – who had always seemed so happy at Princess Christian – was going to be relocated. So we asked our father to find out what was happening." The next day, the father rang Princess Christian officials who initially said, very politely, that the matter could not be discussed. It was a confidential NHS matter. However, eventually the father succeeded in getting an explanation. Princess Christian had been given direct orders to send certain types of patients away to their 'home area' for local councils there to provide accommodation. In this case, the patient had been at Princess Christian for about forty years, seemed to have no living relatives and no one had ever visited him: the only piece of paper that the Hospital had about him was his birth certificate which gave Llandudno as his place of birth. He, therefore, had to be sent there. Although the Hospital staff could not say so formally, they were clearly at least as upset as the schoolgirl by this sudden end of the patient's happy life at Princess Christian: but they had no choice.

Two other people have similar views – Mrs Jill Scott and Dr Adam Skinner. Jill Scott had later founded her own remarkable care home for those with learning difficulties in Tonbridge, The Scotts Project. Jill and her husband, Denis, had lived in Hildenborough since the 1960s and they had got to know a good number of the residents at Princess Christian well. "We would drive down the road to Hildenborough and give them a shout and a wave as they sat on the wall by the shops, watching the world go by and being thoroughly happy," says Jill. She became a Committee Member of the League of Friends and remembers how pleased the Friends were when they were able to provide individual wardrobes in bedrooms. However, when the move towards 'Care in the Community' started, Jill says that she and her husband shared the distress of the Leigh schoolgirls at the brutal and seemingly unplanned way in which long term residents were taken from the only home they had ever known and where their only real friends were. Jill, who herself had a daughter with learning disabilities, emphasized how difficult it always is for people with learning difficulties to make real friendships, other than with people who had similar problems. Dr Adam Skinner, the son of Dr Peter Skinner, the long-time GP at Princess Christian, also wonders about the principle. "I still sometimes see some of the men I knew walking around Tonbridge. They may have lots of friends but I doubt it and I suspect that they had more at Princess Christian and probably more things to do organized for them." Nan Connor, as well as her daughter Nina, have their views too. "By the mid-1980s, I think Princess Christian had become very good," says Nan. "The villa system was working well. The men and women were encouraged to have as much freedom and responsibility as they could cope with. Of course, to have got towards the ideal, we needed more staff, not least to do more training with the 'boys' and 'girls'." Her daughter, Nina, adds, "The residents would have needed more individual space of their own, clothes which they had chosen and so on. If we'd had the money to do all those things, it would have been almost perfect, but they still had a good life." Both mother and daughter also remember instances of men or women being sent off to places where they knew no one. They worried that, someone who had been happy and active in an environment that they knew, might well not cope with a strange place where he knew no one. They remember, too, reading newspaper articles about East Kent where people with learning difficulties were put in b&bs which shut them out in the daytime; and, on a personal basis, Nina remembers one little, elderly lady who had been

Moving Towards the Closure of Princess Christian: 1981–1995

discharged from Princess Christian to a residential home in Hawkenbury on the outskirts of Tunbridge Wells. "She was old and was meant to be retired. But I visited her and found she has been told to clean the Home's ovens. 'Care in the Community' wasn't always as good as the life we helped them have." However, it seems that this type of sudden, traumatic removal and poor care when they reached the outside world probably only occurred at the early stages of the transition and, as will become apparent, caring and detailed plans for the move of patients into the community outlined by David Grant were established more fully as the wind-down of the Hospital continued through the end of the 1980s and into the 1990s.

The Introduction of Charitable Sub-Contractors by the KCC

Having heard about the scale of the task faced by the KCC's Social Services team at the start of 'Care in the Community', it is useful to examine another article[85] about the early days of one of the first voluntary charitable organizations which were employed by KCC to look after the 'residents' who were moved out of Princess Christian. It is important because eventually these charities have become such an integral part of how Kent looks after the people with learning disabilities today. The article comes from April 1987, so roughly two years after the David Grant article. The writer is Bill Griffin, the Project Leader of what was then the relatively new Maidstone Community Mental Handicap Team. There is a grainy photocopy of a photograph of Mr Griffin.

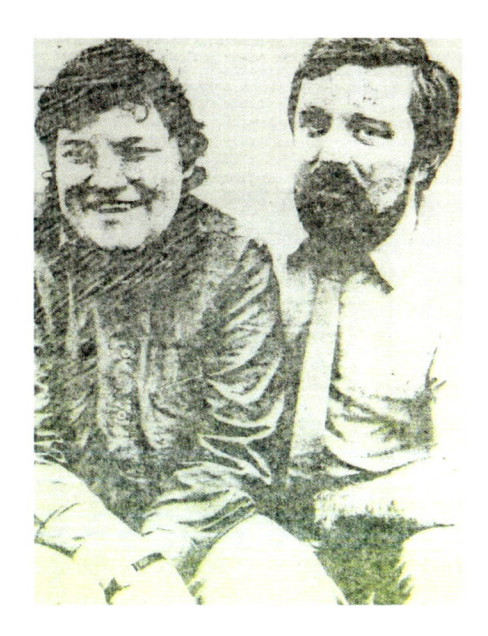

Bill Griffin on right in 1987 –
Project Leader of Maidstone Community
Mental Handicap Team.

Although Bill Griffin's Team had been set up by the Maidstone and Tunbridge Wells NHS Health Authority, it developed gradually into a large, separate, independent charity, mcch, which is described more fully in the second associated book. In 1987, however, it was small. It had sixteen 'clients' – a new term because they were no longer 'residents' – some of whom lived in accommodation rented from the Health Authority or local councils; and some of whom still lived with their relatives – usually their parents. Bill Griffin went on to explain that his next objective was to move thirty-one people who "vary in ability, some having few practical skills and several suffering physical as well as mental disabilities" out of Leybourne Grange and into the community. Following that, he would be moving the remaining thirty-two people out of the old, small Lenham Hospital into six houses which the NHS had acquired. He is absolutely clear that the end of institutional care was vital, even where there are attendant physical or behavioural problems. He is dismissive of the worries of parents who "have never been used to thinking of their son or daughter as being part of their normal peer group. They tend to protect them all the time. If the children are not going to leave home, there is no real pressure to invest time in teaching them skills." Maybe not every parent would have been quite so dogmatic; and his point still can arise in discussions with parents today. He then goes on to give an example of a group of three mentally handicapped people in their thirties – a brother and sister and another man – who had moved into a house together, successfully sharing the upkeep, the cooking, the shopping and the accounts. He explained that one of the men worked for Spadework – a gardening charity, which had originally had its headquarters at Princess Christian Farm. Then the mother of the brother and sister gives her appraisal of the scheme. "There are fors and againsts. I think it gives them a chance to lead more normal lives but there are all sorts of worries that crop up which, if we were dead, we wouldn't know about. All the time that they can cater for themselves, it is all to their advantage, not to ours." Bill Griffin would have agreed. He says, "We are not there to offer a super Valhalla: ordinary life has ups and downs the same as for all of us. We offer the opportunity to do things that the rest of the public take for granted and the responsibility that goes with it." However, it was still early in the ten year programme to run down Leybourne and Princess Christian. The cases quoted applied to those who had relatively mild learning disabilities and the doubts about what would happen later in the journey to those with more complex learning disabilities would still have to be addressed.

Householders' Fears about Mentally Disabled Next Door

Bill Griffin's article has a section which dealt with the fears of ordinary people who would probably be worried about having mentally handicapped people moving next door. Although he does not make the point directly, historically, it was easier in the days of villages when the 'slow' child grew up in the High Street or at the local farm and the people in the parish had known the child all their lives. Then for a hundred and fifty years all sorts of 'mad' people (or people who were unwanted) were shut away from the general public. Now in the 1980s, there were people being released into a world which had little understanding of them as individuals – and a huge range of individuals at that. Bill Griffin approached the problem head on. "Neighbours' fears about having handicapped people next door tend to be based on myths. Residents often fear that their property values will be reduced because of mentally handicapped people next door or that their children will be molested by the newcomers. A lot of people cannot make the distinction between mental illness and mental handicap. Everyone is tarred with the same brush." Bill Griffin concluded, "Research in this country and America has shown that property values were not affected. Nor was there any increase in children being molested." There is probably further research today which supports these two conclusions but it seems not improbable that, even today, neighbours do not initially jump for joy when something similar is proposed in their road. One GP mentioned that some sheltered accommodation provided for several Princess Christian people was on the Hadlow Road in Tonbridge. "The local residents nearby were pretty sniffy – not at all keen", he says.

Funding for the Changes

The last point made by Bill Griffin was how the 'Care in the Community' scheme was to be funded. Where would the money for placing people from Princess Christian Hospital – an NHS organization – into ordinary life, organized by the KCC's Social Services, come from? The cost had to include new accommodation, different types and amounts of oversight and help, as well as more day-care centres and general facilities – all of which meant money from Kent County Council's social services and housing budgets. Bill Cowell had touched on the solution but Bill Griffin explains the practicalities. "The Government worked out that it costs

£11,700 a year to keep someone in a long stay hospital like Princess Christian or Leybourne. If and when that person is discharged that releases that money to provide staff for a year as well as capital investment made by the health authorities."[86] (The fact that Bill Griffin says the money from the NHS budget was only meant to cover a year's worth of care, cannot have greatly pleased any of the Council accountants. Where was the funding to come from for year two or year twenty?) Bill Griffin mentions an additional point. The placing of the funding into an overall pot meant that more money, time and care could be spent on individuals where extra help was particularly needed, while less could be spent where it was not so necessary. But in all cases, he stated, there would be twenty-four hour care available.

The Final Phases of Close Down

There are no records about the speed of the close down at Princess Christian, or of what happened to individual staff. We know that a number of staff retired but we also know in general terms that re-training was done to enable someone who had been a charge nurse at a Princess Christian ward to become a social worker – in some cases continuing to work with people they had known at Princess Christian. For some years, Alexander House was used as a training centre.

The next picture we have of the Princess Christian wind-down comes from a local resident, Mrs Janet Court. Mrs Court had been involved in various senior positions in Kent, first as a KCC Councillor from 1987 to 1994 where she had been Chairman of Kent Schools. She later became a member of the NHS Kent Social Services Committee and then became a member of the West Kent Health Authority from 1992 to 1994. Finally, which included overseeing the closure of Princess Christian, she became Chairman of the Weald of Kent NHS Community Health Trust (WKCHT) which she did until the Hospital was finally wound down around 1994/95. She explains what she found herself and the Community Health Trust doing to implement Government edicts. "Although the general principle of 'Care in the Community' may well have been sensible, it had not initially been clear how the Kent County Council were going to fund the work to completely change the way the Hospital had been looking after its people. Kent County Council Social Services felt they needed all the money that the NHS had been spending on the Hospital, while the NHS said that it was their money and they needed most or all of it for other parts of the Health Service. It took some time to sort out. Eventually, a national policy was agreed. It meant that each 'inmate' who came out of Leybourne Grange or Princess Christian into the wider world – the Social Services world – was given the 'dowry' that you've heard about, from the NHS. When I arrived as Chairman of the Trust, I obviously knew about the general ideas behind 'Care in the Community' – not least from my work in Social Services and in the Health Authority. What we had to do in the Community Health Trust was to see that the people at Princess Christian were going to be well looked after in their new homes – and with their new lives. There had already been steps to wind down the Hospital and most of the larger living quarters on the main site and the Farm were no longer used. The Occupational Therapy building, on the left as you went into the main site, was still much used. By this time there was a sensory room. The residents loved going into the soft ball area. They also loved some flashing disco-type lights that were there. The building had a kitchen which the staff and some of the residents used – although mostly the cooking was done by the men and women in their own villas. On the money side, the 'dowry' enabled Social Services to do a great deal to help the change over and really to look after the people on an individual basis. So I became much involved in the later stages of how 'Care in the Community' actually worked for the Princess Christian people. We had various houses and bungalows in Riding Lane and nearby converted, particularly North and South Cottages on the left of the main entrance; and Barnfield down the road and the house next door. Alexander House, too, was altered and new, purpose-built bungalows were added in the grounds near the entrance. Four bungalows were also built in the grounds of Emily Jackson House in Sevenoaks which had a Day Centre attached; and another group of bungalows and a day centre were built in the grounds of Sherwood House on the Pembury Road in Tunbridge Wells. The future occupants of each house were taken to see their proposed new home a number of times and were allowed to choose the colour schemes for their own rooms and, collectively, decided on the decor and furniture for the living areas, all of which seemed to give them great pleasure. I used to visit all these places to make sure that everything was working well. Each of the houses and bungalows had twenty-four hour carers living in who supervised the cleaning, shopping and cooking arrangements and ensured that residents looked after themselves, including such things as the laundry. Staff accompanied them – where necessary – on trips into the town to shop, to leisure facilities and to doctors and dentists, and generally encouraged them to join in with the local community. The various Day Centres locally had separate specialist staff who organized many activities including pottery, gardening and crafts, as well as sensory sessions for the more disturbed people. These were also attended by people from the local communities with learning disabilities (as we now call them) who were living at home with their families, as well as by some of our residents who still lived in the Hospital. I remember going to a new house and one of our ex-Princess Christian residents said to me, 'do you know that there are lots of different types of bread?' He was thrilled to be out of an institution and into the modern world. Another young woman came to us from Leybourne to be near her parents and had a new bedroom of her own in Alexander House which we had had converted specially. She was really excited and said to me, 'Do you know, I can see horses out of my window. This is going to be my home forever.' The sad thing was that, although that was what we intended at the time, the NHS later sold Alexander House to a developer, just as later they sold the main Princess Christian buildings. The other problem – and it ended up as a major one – was the money which was needed for people coming into the system who had not been at Leybourne or Princess Christian – men and women who had, for example, been living at home. But for various reasons, they now needed accommodation which was suitable for someone with a learning disability. They did not get the £11,700 dowry and the authorities all round Kent found great difficulty in finding somewhere for them to live which was affordable. It did not affect the work I did; but I was conscious that some people with learning disabilities were being housed in bed and breakfast accommodation with little or no help and no real home. It became a public scandal in parts of Kent. However, looking back at Princes Christian, normally the new system did work. I remember very well that the residents always wanted to invite visitors to supper in their new homes. They took it in turns to make the meals and they were absolutely brilliant."

Mrs Court continues, "I believe originally the Farm was established to offer fulfilling and productive work to those living at the hospital, but by the time I was involved, many of the men and women at the Farm came in from the surrounding area – a few by special transport, but most on public buses. Social Services were extremely lucky to find competent agricultural people who also understood and were sympathetic to the problems experienced by their workers. The men and women who came to the Farm looked after a wide range of animals. They bred ducks for sale in the shop and grew vegetables, fruit and plants to sell. Many of the 'workers', as we called them, were part-time but quite a number would be expected to be there every day. What they loved doing most of all was looking after the animals on the Farm.

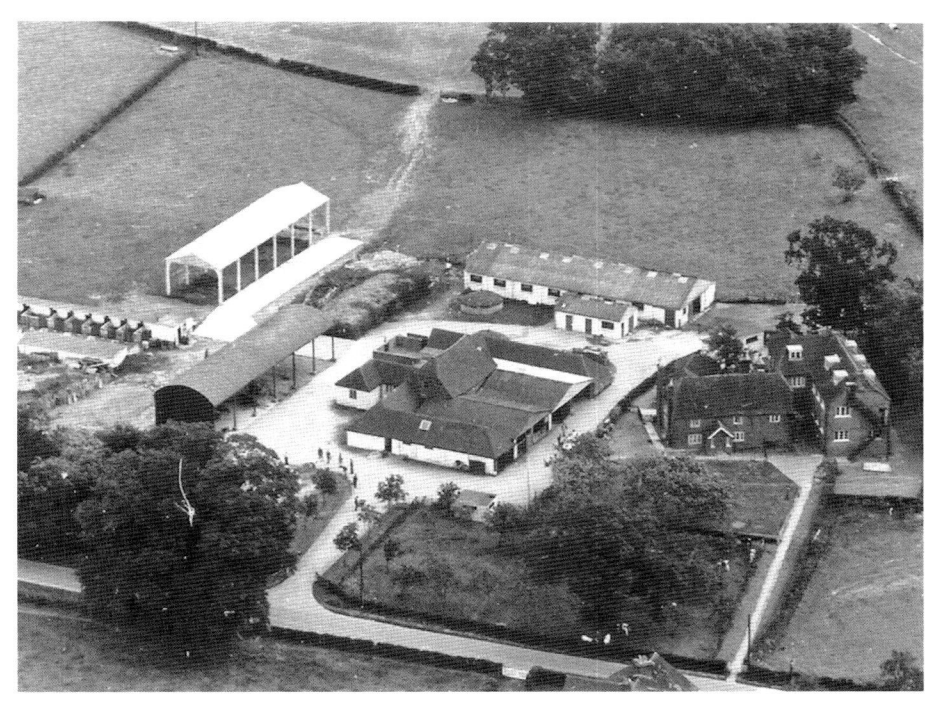

Moving Towards the Closure of Princess Christian: 1981–1995

The Farm. Main building including winter quarters for the cattle in the centre, with the cowshed for milking behind. The piggery is to the left in front of the hay barn. The orchard is to the front/right of the Farm. In the front there is the main Farm House (staff quarters for most of the time) which adjoined the Farm Hostel which housed around ten men.
Photo: from Nan Connor

They groomed and groomed them for hours. The Farm used to enter all the local agricultural shows and usually got the first prizes. What the local farmers thought, I don't know. They didn't have the hours and hours to spend on their animals. And another thing about the animals: You could not impose discipline very easily on those with a learning disability. But if one of them was misbehaving, the punishment could be not being allowed to work with their animals for a time. That worked! But sadly, in the end, Social Services had such a large demand for work at the Farm that not everyone was able to be fitted in there.

"The powers-that-be decided to change the name of what had been called Mental Handicap when I was Chairman of the Community Health Trust. They became 'people with learning difficulties' or, more formally, when the problem was clearly life-long, 'people with learning disabilities'. One parent wrote to me. He was absolutely furious about the change. He said that if his son, who had Down's, was now to be classified as someone 'with learning difficulties', it implied to everyone that it only needed enough time and effort, and his son would improve – which was completely and utterly wrong. He felt that the description 'mental handicap' described accurately his son's life-long problem. I invited him in for a cup of tea and a biscuit and said that, on a personal basis, I very much agreed. We composed a joint letter saying what we thought – but, needless to say, nothing happened. While talking about Down's syndrome, I should mention Tony Langdon-Down. It was his grandfather, Dr John Langdon-Down, who in Victorian times had identified the genetic illness which he called 'mongolism'. When this term went out of fashion in the 1950s and 1960s, it was changed to Down's syndrome in recognition of Dr Down's work. His son, Dr Reginald Langdon-Down (Tony's father) was the Chairman of the Trustees of the Princess Christian Hospital for many years and later its Patron and he did a wonderful job for the first thirty or forty years of the Colony. In his turn, Tony, was a huge supporter as Chairman of the League of Friends of Princess Christian. He attended every single event and meeting, particularly when the Trust was being amalgamated with the Maidstone Community Health Trust and was a most caring man in every way. What was not really public knowledge was that his half-brother, Jack, had Down's syndrome."

The Carers and Wardens who implemented 'Care in the Community' within Princess Christian

Janet Court goes on to emphasize how important it was to have the right level and right quality of support for the men and women who during the late 1980s and early 1990s were being put into the community. This was particularly important because, except in very exceptional circumstances, people with learning difficulties were not formally 'sectioned' and were, therefore, free to leave any accommodation in which they had been placed at any time if they wished to do so. So they were obviously very vulnerable, especially as they could well end up sleeping rough, if they did leave.

One of these carers, or matrons or wardens, was Nancy Vernet who lived in Leigh. For most of her life, Nancy had cared for people, from nursing, to running a playgroup and the Leigh Brownies – "that was for twenty-one years" – to working in a home for battered women with babies. By the 1980s, she had been working for eleven years as a social worker and matron at the Barnardo's boys home at Knotley Hall in Chiddingstone Causeway, near Tonbridge.

Moving Towards the Closure of Princess Christian: 1981–1995

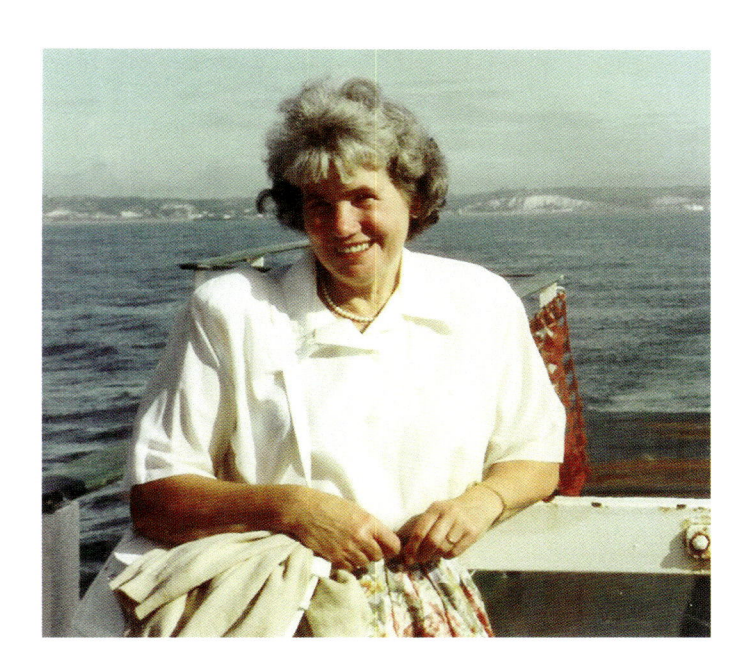

*Nancy Vernet
c. 1990*

After Knotley Hall was wound down, Nancy had started working in an old people's home in Tunbridge Wells: but one day, she saw an advertisement for a vacancy at Princess Christian to work in one of the newly converted, sheltered houses for men in Riding Lane. The kind of care and attention she gave to her eight charges is given in her own words. "In 1986, I saw this ad for a social worker at Princess Christian. It was much nearer home than my job in Tunbridge Wells and it sounded as if it could be more interesting. So I went along and was given the job of Deputy Warden of one of the men's hostel there. The main Princess Christian Hospital was gradually being wound down and the 'boys' and 'girls', as they were still usually called, were being put into sheltered accommodation – usually with people to look after them and help them. My hostel, which was just known as Farm Cottages, was two cottages which had been joined together and I had eight men there to look after. They all worked at the Farm which was just across the road. As far as I remember, lunch was normally provided over the road at the Farm – there was a cook there. But the men organized their own breakfast and we all helped with the evening meal. I got to know the men there very well and still remember them and their circumstances. Some of them had been at Princess Christian for years; and some of them should never have been in an institutional home. It was often that the families felt that the men could not cope. I remember one 'boy', Ron – I guess he was about sixty – who had

The Princess Christian Farm Colony and Hospital 1895–1995

Down's syndrome or whatever you have to call it now. He was absolutely brilliant at ironing: his mother had taught him ages ago. I used to write letters for him to his sister, making it sound as if it was him describing what he had been doing. Then there was one man who had been sent to Princess Christian years before because he had occasional epileptic fits and the parents felt that a Home was the best place for him. (He was rather keen on one of the ladies I also helped to look after sometimes.) One day, he had a fit and I was really worried because it didn't seem to go away like it usually did. So we called the doctor and we tried to revive him; but the doctor said it must have been very severe and he must have died instantly. There was another man (I'd better not say what his name was) whose father came to see him occasionally. The father used to complain about Princess Christian – but he had put his son there. Then there was a man, John, who had elderly parents who lived locally. They were well-to-do but John was still living with us. I suppose they felt they couldn't have coped, particularly as they grew really old. Another John, who came to live in the Hostel, used to help in the Tonbridge market. One day he told them that he was leaving Princess Christian and that he was going to be given a leaving party. We knew he wasn't – he was just moving within our community – but we gave him a party anyway! And there were two old ladies – they were cousins. They had been in the main Princess Christian for years and now they were living in a bungalow opposite the Farm. They were quite OK. They had just been abandoned by their families years ago. Now they were trying to get back to living a normal life.

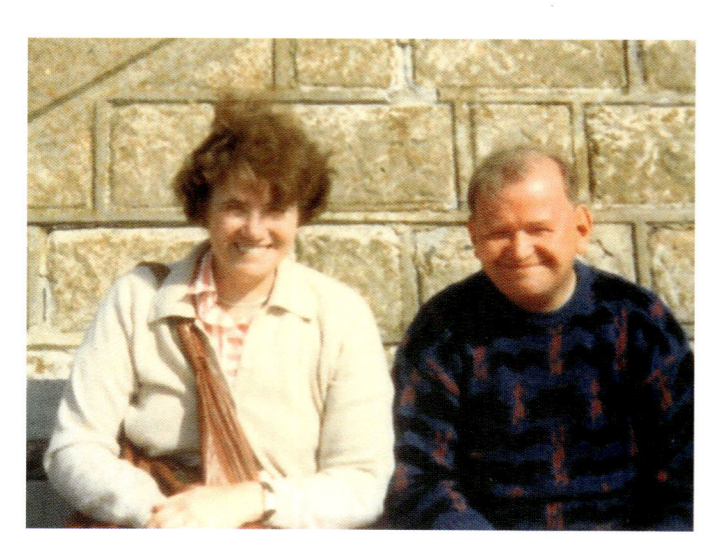

Nancy Vernet, in the late 1980's, with Leslie Goldup. "He was a lovely gentle man: he was almost able to look after himself. It was just that his family couldn't cope for a variety of reasons that we understood. I used to trust him with the keys."
Photo: Nancy Vernet

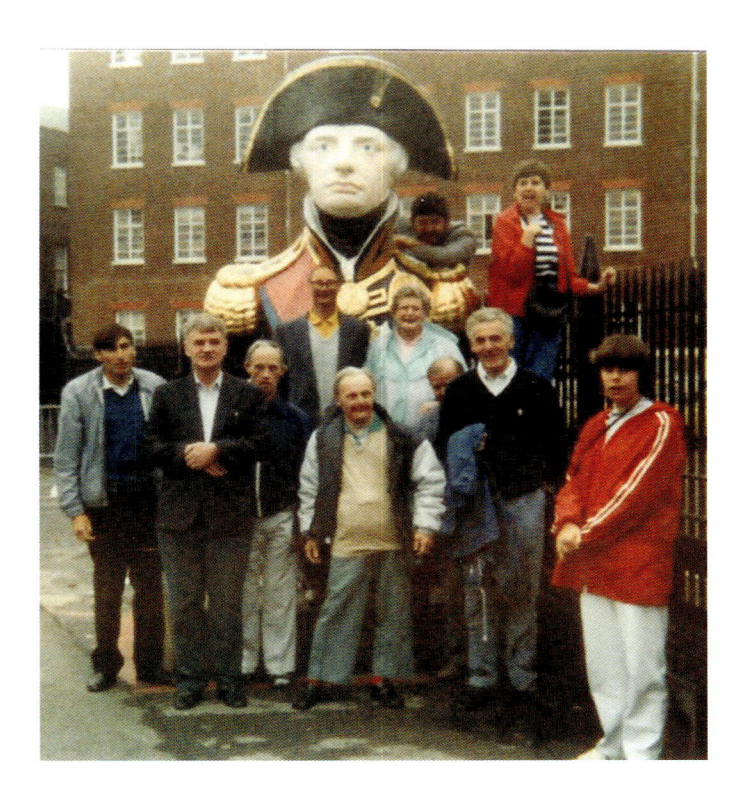

Moving Towards the Closure of Princess Christian: 1981–1995

Nancy Vernet's group on holiday in Portsmouth – with Nelson's statue.
Photo: Nancy Vernet

"Gradually, the powers-that-be tried to get all the men – and women – who had been living at Princess Christian into accommodation where – with suitable help – they could live fairly normal lives within the outside world. It was the right idea, although, as I have said, quite a number of the people at Princess Christian should never have really been there in the first place. The residents had always been looked after very carefully and it continued to be the case when we had the villas and hostels. There were always regular medical check-ups. First, it was Dr Skinner and, in my time, there was his successor – it was usually Dr Brian Glaisher. And there were regular dentist visits. One of our hostel staff always had to be on duty, so I slept in the house opposite once or twice a week for years. The staff would try to give our 'patients' – I'm not quite sure what we called them or were supposed to call them – extra things to do and trips to places they liked. We sometimes took them on holiday – in a caravan – and we went on day trips to Rye and Chichester – places like that."

Nancy continues, "I remember once we went to the Kent County Show. There was a man called Ron – he was from my hostel. He just vanished and everyone was very worried. We rushed around all over the showground but then I remembered that he was very keen on horses, so I set off in that direction. I was just going through the tea tent when he came round the corner – not at all worried. He had been looking at the horses. We tried to give them as normal as life as possible. We used to take them shopping and some of them would go off on their own to do odd jobs. And, where possible, I used to help them keep in touch with their families – as I've said. Sometimes, even after I retired at the end of the 1990s, I still went back there with my husband, Paul, and cooked them all a Sunday lunch or gave one of the men a birthday party."

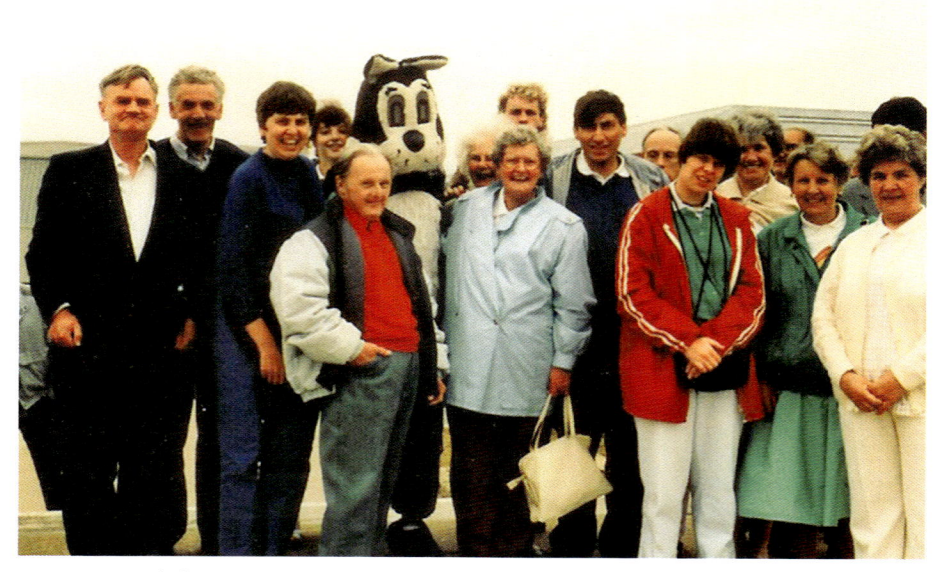

Nancy Vernet's house group on holiday at Butlins.
Photo: Nancy Vernet

Another person who arrived at Princess Christian around 1986/87 as the Hospital was beginning to wind down was Nan Connor's daughter, Nina. For Nina it was really a homecoming. As we have heard earlier, Nina, by now Mrs Brannan, had fond memories of growing up at Princess Christian in what seemed like a family. Everyone knew everyone, "even if we all called each other Mr or Nurse Someone. Never Christian names in those days. And nearly everyone got on with everyone. I was always called 'Mrs Connor's girl'. As children, we had a wonderful time. At Christmas, Mr Pargeter always dressed up as Santa Claus but we also enjoyed all the fêtes and bonfire parties too. It was a real community. So I suppose it was no surprise that I started as a nursing assistant at P.C. before going off to Leybourne to train to be a staff nurse." In 1986, by now fully qualified, Nina was offered the senior post of Ward Manager at Alexander House, one of the 'villas' as they were now being called. She was also in charge of the two bungalows at the end of the drive. "We had twenty-seven gentlemen with 'challenging behaviour', as they called it, in Alexander House and there were five women in one bungalow and five men in the other. The bungalows were for residents who were meant to be getting ready to go out into the community – a sort of half-way house – but, in all honesty, we never really had enough staff to do much to help train them – to prepare them for the wider world. They just had to look after themselves. They got themselves up, did their own cleaning and laundry and so on. All we had time to do was to go over and give them their medicines. Not ideal. But for me this was a high point in my career. I was now in a position to make a difference and try to get away from institutionalization, even though I accepted that this was still an institution in the old sense of the word and that there were strict protocols and rules to follow. The first and most important thing I could do was to ensure that abuse did not take place on this ward. I also adopted a different approach to the old style 'Charge Nurse' whose stereotype was someone with authoritarian and dictatorial leanings, although there were certainly exceptions. I had about ten staff to deal with my twenty-seven 'men' at Alexander House and the two bungalows. The men – the 'gentlemen' as I called them – were nearly all big and strong; and fights used to break out sometimes – not usually with the staff – although I did get knocked down once. We were nearly all women staff – it was difficult to get men to do nursing work – so it could be a bit of a strain at times. We worked in two shifts. Week 1 was Monday, Wednesday, Saturday, Sunday and Week 2 was Tuesday, Thursday and Friday, so alternate weeks you got a full weekend. The shifts were from 7am to 8pm. Overnight there were two what were called 'wake staff'. I looked after one shift and Paddy Griffin – he was a really excellent, far-sighted Charge Nurse – the other. We were meant to have a Staff Nurse and two or three Nursing Assistants each day – although it didn't always happen. I remember that we were grateful to the youngsters, boys and girls, from VSU – the Voluntary Service Unit – who came and entertained the residents. It was good to have a break. One of the first changes I made was to involve the men in the villa in decision making – how they would like their own home run. They formed their own informal discussion groups and fed back the changes they would like to make. There was one very simple thing they requested almost at once – individual teapots on tables, with their own sugar bowls and milk jugs so they controlled the pouring of their tea, rather than the staff walking around with a big teapot. We spent time raising money at the annual fête and coffee mornings to help fund new, non-regulation china. After these events, there would be much excitement, counting our takings. Then, together we spent time individualizing each person's own space. Shelves were put up for their books. Some of the men enjoyed music and chose to buy themselves tape players. Others wanted their own TV – previously there had been one main TV room for everyone on the ward, with up to thirty patients at any one time, all watching the channel that would be chosen by a staff member. Photographs were put in frames by their beds. Old sheets and blankets were discarded and replaced with duvets and covers of their own choice. This all took time and needed money which we had to raise ourselves. But the atmosphere among the staff and patients was one of excitement and they all enjoyed working towards the next goal. I had felt concern that some of the older staff members would be resentful of these changes but, on the whole, the ideas were positively embraced and I was very lucky to have Paddy as my deputy. There was competition over who could have the next good idea. The state of the building was very run down. The toilets and bathrooms were well below standard and everything was in need of attention. I repeatedly tried to get the management – who were all at Leybourne if it had anything to do with money – to do something. Eventually a man came over. He looked around and said 'I don't know how anyone who has pride in their work could live in such a mess'. I was extremely cross. AND we didn't get any money. I guess by this time they hadn't got any money, particularly for buildings which were soon to be wound down. But he was not very tactful! Unfortunately, all was not plain sailing, The 'challenging behaviour' increased. I was at a loss to understand this as I naively thought that, as the home environment improved, so would their behaviours. Our aim – it was about 1988/89 and quite a number of the other men and women residents had been already re-housed – was to get our 'gentlemen' ready to look after themselves in the wider world, so it was not ideal that things were actually getting worse. When the problems increased, I was lucky that they found a really good psychologist, Cecille Gorney, who, over the next year, gave us advice. She said it was happening because the men had never been given much freedom and choice before – they had always been led closely by staff. She positively encouraged the changes and stayed with me for a year, working alongside the ward staff to help acclimatize the men to their new, changing conditions and what would soon be their new lives."

A local couple told a story which confirmed the problems that could arise when changes were introduced. At one point later in the Princess Christian story, the Hospital management, wanting to make the atmosphere more informal, issued an edict that staff should not wear uniforms. However, the 'boys' and 'girls' were upset. So the late Nurse Ursula Taylor, one of the senior staff at Glen House, decided off her own bat to buy white shirts and matching navy blue cardigans for all her staff. Nina confirms that her 'boys' at Alexander House did not like the change, so she and her colleagues there continued to wear uniforms, including the nurse's belt, for weekdays but not at weekends. There was much the same reaction when another edict came down in the later 1980s: all staff from now on had to be known by their Christian names. For most of the 'boys' and 'girls' this was unsettling. It did not seem natural. For ten or twenty years, they had called the staff 'Nurse Somebody' or Mr Brown. "So, we did not enforce the rule but neither did we object if we were called by our Christian name," Nina explained. "There was one example of institutional behaviour that I particularly remember which summarizes the old style and what we were now trying to introduce. One morning I was in the dormitories opening windows, when I came across two men who would not normally have been on the ward at this time. They were in the middle of a sexual act. I knew both men well and they were horrified to see me. I said, 'sorry, excuse me' and quickly left, closing the door behind me. A few minutes later they returned to the lounge. They appeared embarrassed and nervous as to what might happen next. In previous years and under the old type of management, such behaviour would have had bad consequences. It was not unknown following an incident such as this, for a patient to be humiliated by a member of staff, privately and publicly, and to have their meagre 'pocket money', as it was called at the time, withdrawn. I purposely spoke to them in a normal manner. I did not refer to the incident. Having worked with the men for several years, I did not feel that either party was being abused and I felt that they were both consenting adults. At the time, sexual relationships were not approved of in institutions, but staff were aware that some patients were sexually active. It was a matter of staff deciding if either party was not consenting. We had been given an information folder by one of the agencies involved with the process of helping the patients with the transition to small community homes. These included a pamphlet which explained that people with a learning disability have the same rights as the rest of the community – including the right to normal sexual activity. My aim was to gradually reduce fear and embarrassment about it. One quote in the pamphlet said: 'People with a disability have the same sexual needs as people without handicaps. However, carers and staff must ensure that people are free from sexual abuse or exploitation'. Most of the men undoubtedly had various problems but they were always aware of what was going on. Several of them were good mimics. One used to watch me doing things at the end of my shift, writing up my notes and telephoning Paddy about the hand-over to the next shift and so on – and then he'd pretend to be me. He would put on my nurse's belt and write away and pick up the phone and do an imitation of me talking to Paddy. In their own way, they took in everything.

"Although we were officially responsible to the Head of Nursing at the Hospital, we were very lucky that we were also really well supported by the Hildenborough GP's practice. I remember Dr Brian Glaisher who came up on a regular basis but also if there was something special or difficult. As I mentioned earlier, we had drug charts for all the men and we were always discussing how maybe we could cut back the dose for one or another of the men. They were certainly not drugged up to keep them quiet. We'd never have done that. In due course, sheltered accommodation with various different degrees of help was found for all our men. It must have been in 1989 when all my people in Alexander House and the two bungalows had moved out and I spent about six months on the management side. My mum stayed on even after me but I hope that what I did over the three or four years at Alexander House was sensible and a change for the better."

Nina Brannan has lucidly explained the staff's attitude to sexual activity. So it is worth mentioning the comment of a local farmer who had been in the area for over forty years and knew about Princess Christian Hospital, although as an outsider. He said, almost in passing, "everyone knew that the 'girls' at Glen House were on the pill." He knew no more than "everyone knew it" – or assumed it. However, this rumour is denied by Nan Connor who for so many years had overseen Glen House, including dispensing all the medicines given to the 'girls'. "As far as I know, 'the pill' was never given to any of my 'girls'. Sometimes romantic attachments were formed between the women and the men but then it was the staff's job to see that things didn't go too far. But I'm clear the rumour was wrong."

Another local person, who was a nursing assistant or auxiliary nurse, looked mainly after the men. She was at Princess Christian for twenty-two years from 1980 to 2002 and in that time she saw Princess Christian change from being a Hospital – appreciated by those who lived there – to the start of a 'Villa' system – which she felt worked really well. And following that, she saw the coming of the outside contractors who were employed by Kent County Council to provide 'Care in the Community.' At the start of her

Moving Towards the Closure of Princess Christian: 1981–1995

career in 1978, she had worked at Pembury Hospital, near Tunbridge Wells but went to Princess Christian Hospital in 1980, where she was nearer her home and family. She often did the night shifts because this allowed her to look after her children during the day. She worked mainly looking after the men at the Farm Villa – first when it was down beside the Farm itself and then when the Villa was moved into what had been the Admin Building: but she also sometimes looked after the men in Alexander House, or the Oast House, or the Hostel (the house next to the Farm). Occasionally, too, she looked after the women up at Glen House. Whenever one of the other carers was off sick or had had some emergency, she would get a call at the last minute just as she and her husband were going out for the evening to ask if she could do the shift that night. Her husband was used to it and he'd tell her to go. And she went because she loved the job and the people she looked after. She says, half jokingly, that naturally there were individuals amongst those she looked after who were a bit more difficult than the rest; but that only made her try particularly hard to help them. But the job was so rewarding. Her children were regular visitors and one daughter trained to become a mental health nurse. The job meant that she was in sole charge of often twenty eight men all by herself from eight at night until seven in the morning. The only supervision would be the charge nurse who would come round, usually once in the night. Every morning when the men got up, those who were able to, made their own beds. If you were able to make your bed, you felt very superior to those who couldn't. There were no major disasters over the years but one problem was that thunder and lightning quite often made the fire alarms go off. So all the residents had to be woken up – they were not always very keen – and they had to be assembled at the fire point where they had a roll call. Several times there was one particular man missing and she'd find that he had gone back to his room to make his bed! She agreed that the initial period of closing the Hospital could produce very unfortunate cases. "Unless the resident had lived in the area paid for by Tunbridge Wells Health Authority or at the least in West Kent, they just got sent off somewhere in the country, away from all the people they had lived with, often for twenty or even forty years. It was not good. There are still some old Princess Christian residents in Tonbridge and I still see them and get a hug. But they are getting old and soon there won't be any left. There is one man – he's eighty-four now – whom I looked after for all the twenty-two years I was at Princess Christian. When they moved the men and women down to Tonbridge, I guess that they might have been a bit surprised to start with but I think they got used to the idea fairly soon, particularly as a good number of their carers were initially people who had looked after them at Princess Christian and where in a good number of cases they were in accommodation with others they had lived with at Princess Christian." She does not think that if you asked these elderly men nowadays whether they preferred Princess Christian or where they were today, any of them could remember that far back. By the end of the 1980s, the nurse felt that conditions for the 'residents' and staff – but particularly the 'residents' who she felt were the most important – had improved from the time she had joined ten years before, particularly with the development of its own villa system. "By 1990, the whole atmosphere could be more relaxed. The staff were not just custodians." It was community care but under the Princess Christian system, with the residents living with people they knew, in a place they knew and in an area which they knew; and which understood them. She is proud to have been one of the people who helped set up this new Villa system. She took her residents on holidays, both in England and abroad – with only one other nurse – and she felt her reward was seeing how much they enjoyed themselves. She still thinks that the system of community homes within Princess Christian was "really good". However, when the Kent County Council started using outside care providers, she started to suspect that the attitude towards the residents was beginning to change. She became employed by one of the new charities doing the work for Kent County Council Social Services (although she was able to retain her NHS terms and conditions). She says she felt that many of the new staff were not likely to be as dedicated as the old Princess Christian staff had been – many of whom had been at Princess Christian for even longer than she had been. She feels strongly that under the new system of 'Care in the Community' – delivered by outside contractors – there was not and could not really be the close relationships that you used to have between Princess Christian staff and its 'residents'. There were also instances when she was disgusted by the attitudes of her new bosses in the outside contractors. Eventually, she was so disillusioned that she took early retirement at 55 in 2002.

Spadework

It is often thought that Spadework, which over the last thirty years has done excellent work in training and giving an occupation to people with learning disabilities, was part of Princess Christian. This was never the case and, indeed, the start of Spadework in 1984 came because a number of parents locally, who had children with learning difficulties, were dissatisfied with the lack of stimulation that they felt was provided for their children by Social Services. They, therefore, started their own charity and persuaded the Princess Christian management to let them have an overgrown corner of the Farm as their first headquarters. The full story of Spadework and its current role is given in the second, associated book, "Couldn't You Just Call Me John."

The Final Farewell Party

Right towards the end of its life, probably in 1993 or 1994, there was a final farewell party. Rosemary Tidby was and still is an NHS community nurse. She used to refer some of her young men to the Farm which she visited quite often. Over the years she had got to know some of the staff at the Hospital itself and was invited to the party. "It was held in the big hall which was all decorated. But it was all very sad. There was hardly anyone there. I suppose nearly all, if not all, the 'boys' and 'girls' had been relocated and it was probably thought untactful to invite them back. And I guess many of the younger staff had moved on too. So there was just a few staff who were retiring and a few outsiders, like me. It wasn't at all like the family it had always been. As I say, all rather sad." Nan Connor, told of the party many years later, says that no one told her about it. Although she had retired (after thirty-five years), she only lived down the road. "Obviously, it was arranged by people who didn't really know about the real Princess Christian."

CHAPTER 5

Coda: What Happened to The Buildings; and to the 'Boys' and 'Girls'?

The Main Site

In the mid-1990s, the main Princess Christian site was sold by the NHS to Berkeley Homes. Glen House, as a Grade II listed building, had to be retained by Berkeley Homes, but they suggested to the Tonbridge & Malling Borough Council Planners that all the other buildings were so old or ill-built that they should be demolished. The Borough Council accepted this assessment but laid down two principal conditions. There had to be some apartments/smaller homes; and the 1904 Clough Williams-Ellis design for the pseudo-oast house must be rebuilt using the original plans. The result was thirty-one homes in an estate called Hilden Brook Farm.[87] The development was, and is, still considered well laid out and to fit in well with local Kentish styles, even if the new homeowners raised a considerable number of complaints about the quality of the finish to the buildings. The first homes were occupied at the start of 1999 and the final ones – the rebuilt Oast House – two years later. A plaque to the Langdon-Down family which had been unveiled by Ruth Langdon-Down in 1924 was repositioned as the back of a seat near the entrance. However, recently an irony has surfaced. A local was chatting to the brickie who had erected the seat. The brickie said the stone was not the original one. It had disintegrated. So they had cobbled together a replacement!

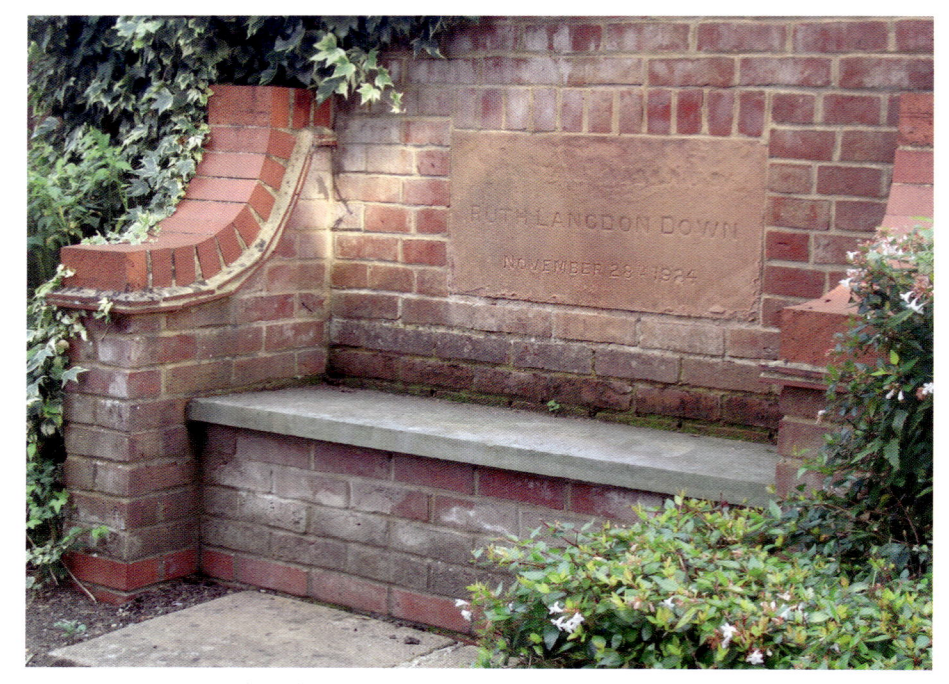

Stone seat now outside Hilden Brook Farm estate.
Photo: Anna Rowley

Glen House

However, there were difficulties about the renovation of Glen House. After Berkeley Homes had undertaken what they claimed was a full modernization, the house was sold to Richard and Julie Ingram in 1999 with ten and a half acres of land. It became clear that the renovations had been done very badly, or not at all, and eventually the Ingrams took Berkeley Homes to the High Court – winning the case. After four years the actual restoration of Glen House was finished, including around sixty new made-to-measure windows. The work had been overseen by inspectors to ensure the workmanship was up to Grade II listing standards and finally the Ingram family could live in the house without twenty or thirty workmen with them. The Ingrams even had the bell replaced in the 'clocktower' which had been taken away sometime over the past fifty years. A large conservatory was also added at the eastern end which one local resident said was considerably larger than his three bedroom house. At the end of 2014, the Ingrams put this by now absolutely beautiful house up for sale.

Coda: What Happened to the Buildings; and to the 'Boys' and 'Girls'?

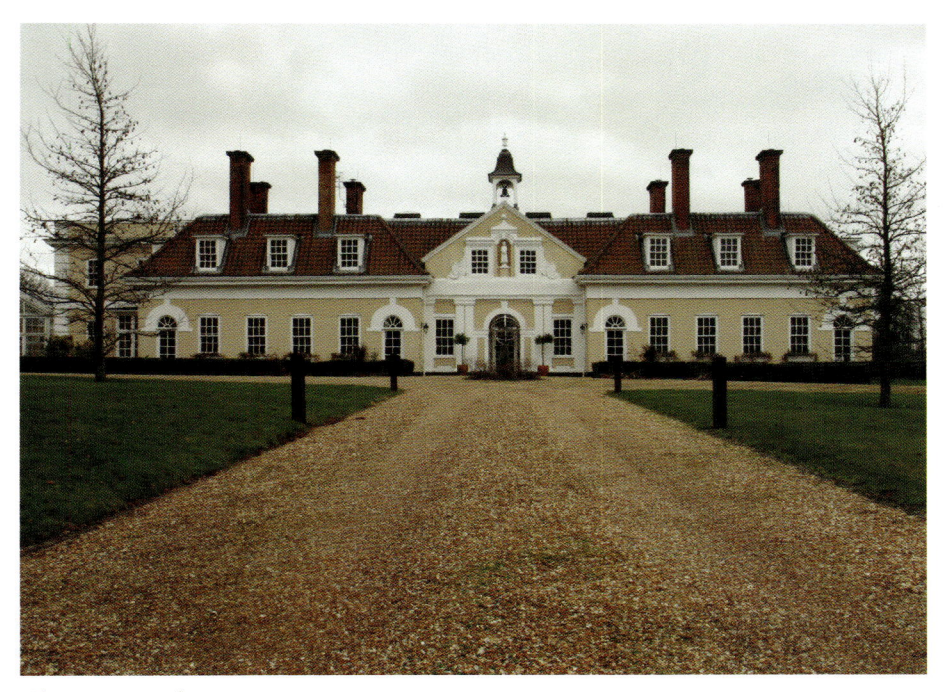

Glen House today.

Photo: Juliet Rowley

Alexander House

Alexander House also had its problems. One local resident says that the house had never been owned by the NHS. A trust connected to the Langdon-Down family (or perhaps to the National Association) had apparently leased out the house and land rent-free to the NHS but only on the basis that it was used for those with learning disabilities. After the final closure of the main Hospital in the mid-1990s, the NHS seems to have used the house as some sort of respite home for people with learning difficulties; and at a later stage at least the downstairs was used as an NHS training centre. One person remembers attending a course there in 2005 or 2006 to be told about the new Mental Capacity Act. At some stage fairly soon after this, the NHS sold the building and most of the grounds to a developer on the basis that it would continue to be used for some kind of learning disability/mental health purpose. Perhaps, not surprisingly, the developer did not seem to have that kind of objective in mind and he applied for a change of use. He wished to build a housing estate.

The Princess Christian Farm Colony and Hospital 1895–1995

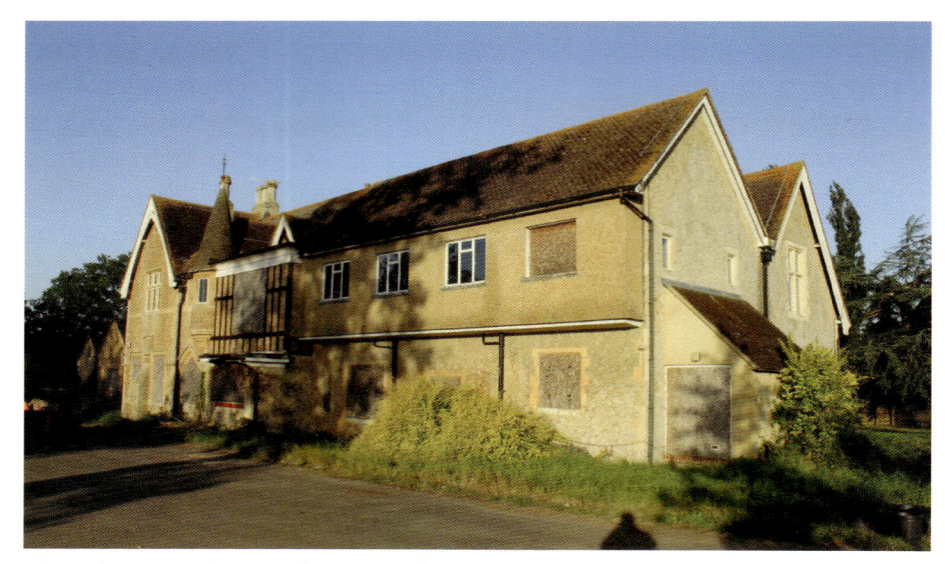

Alexander House in 2012, having just been bought by Mark and Liz Smith, after it had been sold by the NHS around 2008.
Photo: Mark and Liz Smith

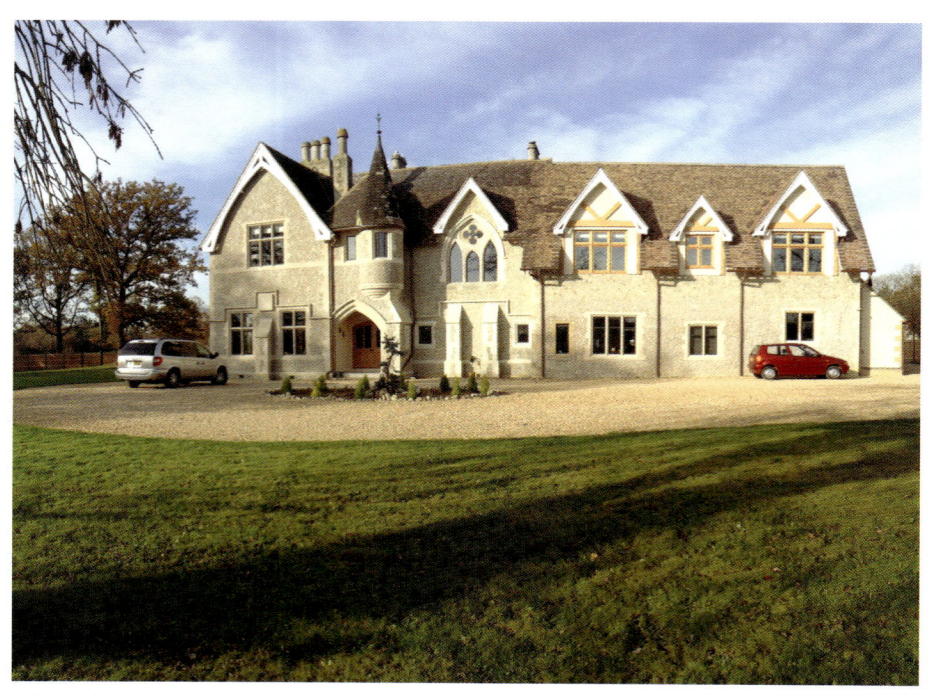

Alexander House in 2014 now rebuilt by Mark and Liz Smith.
Photo: Mark and Liz Smith

Coda: What Happened to the Buildings; and to the 'Boys' and 'Girls'?

Permission was refused. After the house and grounds had lain derelict for a number of years, a local resident, Mr Stuart Howard, who lived at The Vines and was not keen on the possibility of an estate at the end of his garden, bought the house and most of the land from the developer. At this point the building was in a very run down state with the windows boarded up and with rotting old NHS mattresses on the floors upstairs.

Mr Howard removed the worst of the rubbish from inside and then, in 2012, sold the house to Mark and Liz Smith. The Smiths found themselves with a property which had to be completely gutted and modernized. They decided to restore the house to what it had been in 1920, including making good the damage caused by the fire in the early 1960s which had destroyed the middle of the front upstairs of the house. When the repairs had been undertaken in the 1960s, they had been done in the least expensive way possible and had destroyed the mid-Victorian look of the building. After a year of intensive work, the house had been dramatically redone and now resembles the house as it was when it was used by Reginald Langdon-Down in the first part of the 20th century – but with a large number of mod cons.

Hadlow College and the Farm

However, there was one local scheme on the original Farm Colony site that did continue to look after the type of men and women who had been catered for over the last ninety years – the Princess Christian Farm itself and an expanded Farm Shop. After some indecision, the Kent County Council allowed Hadlow College to take over the Farm on a ninety-nine year lease from 2009 at a modest rent. There were conditions, however, particularly the overarching one that people with learning difficulties should continue to be trained on the Farm site.

The People's Memories and Views from the Local Community

However, much more important than what happened to the buildings – even if they had been built with such care, often by the 'boys' themselves, and with such fund raising efforts – was what was happening to the range of people who were looked after at Princess Christian.

The aim of the Hospital had always been to make those at Princess Christian feel they were part of the community as far as was possible; and the management of the Hospital had supported the principle behind 'Care in the

Community' long before it became an active Government policy. Many local residents witnessed the changes over the fifty years after the Second World War and have fond memories of that era. Nancy Ashwell who lived at The Cottage in Riding Lane when she was a girl from the mid-1930s to the early 1950s, remembers the 'boys' and 'girls' walking down Riding Lane in a crocodile, two by two holding hands – although the men and women were always separate. This description is echoed by many other Hildenborough residents – several adding that sometimes the outside man or woman would hold a rope which would stretch from the front to the back of the crocodile. Mrs Monica Cecil remembers that in the 1960s and 1970s during the school holidays, Princess Christian people provided magnificent Meals on Wheels food which was then delivered by the WRVS drivers; and in the 1980s several Princess Christian men used to come to the Hildenborough Church fairly regularly. "One, whose name I think was Norman, came there early to help distribute the hymn books and prayer books. I still see him about in Tonbridge from time to time." Many other Hildenborough residents remember the 'colonists' walking by themselves down to the shops in Hildenborough to spend their pocket money or just for a walk and a chat with the locals. Everyone thought of them as occasionally in need of a bit of help, but essentially kind and gentle. Pat and Anne Davies, who lived almost next door to Princess Christian, saw all the changes. They not only knew many of the residents but see several of them in Tonbridge today, twenty-five years later. "I remember Alan, a fair-haired man, probably fortyish who always greeted every car with a huge thumbs up and a shout of 'Wotcha mate' as he walked between The Colony and the Farm on the footpath," says Pat, "but if you got close to him he was painfully shy and used to partially cover up his face. Then there was Sid – he was a Jeremy Corbyn lookalike – who would walk a bit, then stop and think, then start again and so on, all the time repeating the same thing over and over again. Then there was another man, whose name I've forgotten who used to call me 'the bird on a bike' because I used to whistle to him as I rode my bike to get the commuter train at Hildenborough station. And I still see a man, Smithy, and a friend of his, whose name I've forgotten, in Tonbridge. Smithy was a regular at the PC fêtes and, because he had a very square build, he used to be the anchor for the tug-of-war team."

There is no consensus about whether life was better for the men and women when they lived at Princess Christian or when they became part of Care in the Community. Brian and Gillian Taylor, remember one of the 'boys' was very upset when he was moved into sheltered housing in

Coda: What Happened to the Buildings; and to the 'Boys' and 'Girls'?

Tonbridge. They still see him to wave to but they, too, have not felt that they can ask him how he feels nowadays, twenty-five years later. Joy Dolling and her husband, Howard, recall seeing a man they had known at Princess Christian in Bexhill when they were driving through to a meeting. "He had what you'd nowadays call cerebral palsy but we just called it being a spastic – there was no shame in the word. When we saw him, he seemed to be wandering about but we couldn't stop in the traffic and ask him how he was. But we did wonder if he was happy." Once the author was talking with a man who is chairman of a large group which runs old people's homes and who had occasion to visit a home for men with learning disabilities just outside his own Sevenoaks/Tonbridge area. It was purpose built; it had very well-equipped individual flats for the six or so men; and there was a caring warden, with well-made communal meals if and when the residents wanted them. As he went into the home, he was approached by one of the men who said that he used to live a Princess Christian "which was much better than here." However, it would only be fair to add that when the visitor had first entered the house, the resident had hurried up to him and asked, "Do you come from Tonbridge – I know you." The warden leant over and whispered, "Don't worry. He says that to everybody." So it is difficult to say for certain that the former Princess Christian resident had really liked Princess Christian quite as much as he said.

However, definite support for the situation as it is today comes from yet another Hildenborough resident who knew one of the younger men at Princess Christian well and whom he still meets quite often. The Hildenborough resident has no doubt that, however well the 'boys' and 'girls' were looked after at Princess Christian, the man he knows certainly prefers leading his own independent life. This kind of positive view of Care in the Community was echoed by Rosemary Tidley, the very experienced Community Learning Disability Nurse, who remembered the Princess Christian Hospital in the early 1990s, as well as the Princess Christian Farm. She thought the Hospital had given good care by the standards of its time but things had clearly moved on and the system was so much better today. She also felt the Farm was and still is a great resource for the area. "I used to find that if I had what you used to call a 'naughty boy', I would suggest that he tried to get a place at the Farm. It could be – and still is – wonderful for them and they nearly all not only enjoy themselves but get a lot out of it. It meant and it still means that they are actually DOING something, rather than just sitting around back in their room."

I talked with a very knowledgeable man who had a brother with Down's syndrome. The brother had spent all his early life in Leybourne Grange. The brother, who was never able to talk, was very happy at the hospital, with friends who had been with him for twenty years and staff whom he liked. When plans for Care in the Community were mooted, the man's father was passionately against the idea. In spite of the father's opposition, the son was put into sheltered housing. However, his closest friends from the mental hospital went with him and the sheltered accommodation was well managed and in a sensible location. Eventually, the father accepted that the outcome was a huge success – for everyone. Another positive example of moving people out of a psychiatric hospital into sheltered accommodation comes from Penny Southern, the current KCC Director of Learning Disabilities and Mental Health. Thirty years ago, she arrived in Kent to work at Leybourne Grange Hospital. She had started as a Care Assistant in the East Midlands before moving to Devon to help wind down a psychiatric hospital there. Her new job was to ensure that people leaving Leybourne were found good quality, suitable accommodation – where possible with people they knew. It was relatively easy where the person concerned had been born fairly locally or at least in Kent. However, as we have seen, where this was not the case, they had to be sent to their 'Place of Origin'. Penny had one couple who had lived together at Leybourne for over ten years. Unfortunately, bureaucratically, they had two places of origin – one in Folkestone (in Kent) and one in Hastings (in East Sussex). They were to be given two different flats in the two towns. However, Penny managed to get the Kent man's funding transferred to the East Sussex authorities and a flat for two was found for them in Hastings.

Bill Richardson and Ron Wood, who had lived all their lives near Princess Christian, represent the views of nearly everyone in Hildenborough who have talked about the Hospital (although both men mention that it was never called a hospital by locals. It was usually called 'The Colony' or Princess Christian or occasionally 'The Farm' or 'Princess Christian Farm' or 'PC' or very occasionally 'PCH'.) The men and women were always called the 'boys' and the 'girls' – whatever their ages – although it was always difficult to know just how old they were. The 'boys' and 'girls' were always kept segregated. However, as Bill says, "human nature being what it is, we did hear that occasionally friendly relations were formed. They got round the regulations somehow." Bill and Ron also recall that one of their earliest memories in the 1940s onwards was "to see the separate column of up to fifty boys or girls – they were always separate – walking down the road two-by-two, hand-in-hand in a crocodile." After Ron left school in the mid-1950s, he had gone to

Coda: What Happened to the Buildings; and to the 'Boys' and 'Girls'?

work at Great Forge Farm and at Mr Hubble's Farm, both further down Riding Lane. He was paid a shilling an hour to help in the fields or in the market garden. "There was really only one labourer on each farm and so when there was a busy period – the harvest and times like that – they used to hire in the 'boys' from the Colony. The farmers paid half a crown an hour which went to the Colony, I suppose," says Ron, "but it did seem a bit rough on me when I got less than half that. However, if you complained, you got given the less willing 'boys'. And, anyway, they didn't always do a very good job. The trick was to offer them a packet of Woodbines – that got them really keen." There were things for the 'girls' to do as well. Ron remembers, "In the 1960s my aunt, Wynne Woodgate (now passed on) used to work at the laundry and in the needlework part of The Colony to help the 'girls' learn what to do."

Like nearly all the local residents both men remember the social side too. "The club had its own bar as well as various games", says Bill. "And there were very cheerful dances there. They were often organized and attended by VSU – the Voluntary Service Unit. The 'boys' and 'girls' used to wait outside each week for the VSU bus to arrive. My brother used to go along to help, too, and there were quite a few evening occasions when the adult helpers got a bit the worse for wear. I remember once or twice I had to run people home in my car. And there was a very well organized firework display each year." Both men reckon, too, that the League of Friends was an excellent organization. "They raised large amounts of money to get extra things for the 'colonists', as well as helping guide the whole organization in sensible ways. Mr Tony Langdon-Down was a huge supporter for many years." Bill feels strongly that it was (and is) wrong to characterize all the 'boys' and the 'girls' as 'mentally retarded' or whatever description was (and is) given to them. "They may all of them have had problems of looking after themselves in the outside world without help," he says, "but they were all different when you got to know them. One, Jock, was certainly not at all slow. He was somewhat deformed and his family – who were rich – thought that he would be better off at Princess Christian. The parents used to come and see him two or three times a year, and once every year they would take him to the tailors in Tonbridge to have a new suit – or suits – made for him. (His old ones were passed on to the other 'colonists'.) There were several like that. The families just felt that they couldn't cope; and there were other 'boys' and 'girls' there who certainly weren't stupid – they just had a very narrow interest and couldn't understand anything else. There was Richard who could tell you absolutely everything about steam trains. And there was another man who used to collect wood because he said he wanted to make rabbit hutches. He'd always be coming in to the yard of a friend of mine just off Riding Lane who made sheds. And I used to see him coming out of Baltic Sawmills in Tonbridge, down by the river, with bits of wood everywhere – sticking out of his pockets and everywhere. I never knew whether he made any rabbit hutches!" Some of the 'colonists' were re-housed in Hildenborough and Tonbridge. Both Ron and Bill say that they still see some of the 'boys' they knew back in the 1970s and 1980s in Tonbridge. "But I still think that winding up Princess Christian in the way that they did was a mistake," says Bill.

Bob Duffin, who had known Princess Christian since his childhood in the 1930s, approaches the subject of the closure from a slightly different viewpoint. Although he was fond of the 'boys' and 'girls' and thought that the staff treated them well, his job – a delivery driver mainly to hospitals – took him to a number of the large asylums for the mentally ill. He particularly remembers the Epsom lunatic asylum as being a terrible place; and once he went to the mental hospital at Redhill. "Round the front was OK but I and my mate, Eric Spender, went round the back. There were lots of men penned into a metal enclosure – just like sheep. It was horrible. I shall never forget it. They were being treated like animals by ignorant members of the stores staff. So when I heard that all the mental hospitals were being wound up, I was glad. But that didn't include Princess Christian. I didn't want Princess Christian closed." It is particularly ironic that the Redhill Mental Hospital was where Dr John Langdon-Down had started his career of reforms for the care of his patients over a hundred years earlier. The description of Redhill Hospital by Bob Duffin is echoed by a description of many other old lunatic asylums all round the country. For example, there was Exminster Hospital in Devon in the same period, which housed one thousand four hundred inmates in a building designed for four hundred and forty; and where inmates were chained together in groups of three to discourage escape attempts.[88] More locally, there was Oakwood Mental Hospital at Barming. Although there were no scandals, several local people had relatives who, even as late as the 1970/80s, were sectioned there. They have described an appallingly depressing place, hugely out-of-date with corridors that went on for miles and with patients screaming. However hard the staff worked, it was not an environment likely to help the patients recover. It was reports of places such as these that led Parliament to pass laws which led to the closure of all mental institutions, including the many which were unacceptable but also the Princess Christian Hospital.

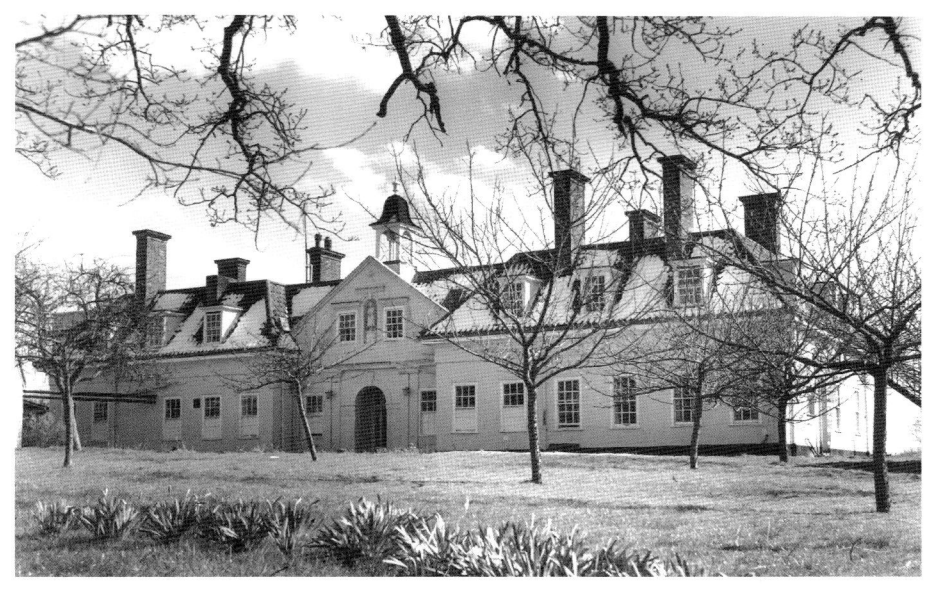

Coda: What Happened to the Buildings; and to the 'Boys' and 'Girls'?

Glen House as it was towards the end of its life.
© *The Kent & Sussex Courier, 21 April 1978*

Perhaps one of the most interesting view from a local came from the late Tony Langdon-Down. As someone so closely involved since his childhood, his views were likely to be constructive. The thoughts come in a Spotlight article in 1984. He says that the authorities should "continue to think about the extent 'normalization' could go without endangering the very strengths that Princess Christian and other pioneer hospitals had achieved in the past." This view could be seen just as an old-timer defending the system which his father had set up eighty years before, following his grandfather's ideals. However, his idea was more perceptive than that. The Princess Christian Hospital had wanted to have its residents more able to live in mainstream life. In the 1980s it had set up villas and cottages for those who were able to live more independently, although help was available when needed. Maybe the system did not have the money to buy up more houses or have more staff but in essence was not Tony Langdon-Down saying that, although more of the people at Princess Christian could and should leave and become part of the outside world, there would always be the need for more specialist help and specialist accommodation for those who were never going to be able to look after themselves by themselves? And was he perhaps also saying that a good proportion of people with learning difficulties would always be best served in a home with their friends around them? 'Normalization' or sometimes just placing them in the wider world could go too far. This doubt is shared by Dr Adam Skinner, who – after his gardening job at Princess Christian – became a local GP. In his own GP practice in Westerham, he has dealt with a good number of children and adults with learning difficulties. He feels that it is not automatically better to place them all in flats on their own, with occasional advice but not necessarily any companionship or any easy way to be part of the community. However, the debate about whether it was a good idea to wind down The Princess Christian Hospital and whether it was always done sensitively will never be entirely resolved.

What was to be the last view about 'before' and 'after' Care in the Community came from Roger Gibson, the now retired Chief Executive of Pepenbury, a large unit for people with a wide variety of learning disabilities at Pembury, near Tunbridge Wells. "I have known many people who have initially lived in a community like the old Princess Christian Hospital or our main facility here at Pepenbury. Where possible, we have helped them to go out to live in their own independent sheltered units or their own flats. And, however happy they were at Princess Christian or in our community, not one of them would prefer to be back. They like to be out in the real world."

I was aiming to end the book on this positive note. It has been told to me by a man I trusted and liked. However, I have recently been finishing a companion book about how people who are like those at Princess Christian are supported today. The book is called 'Couldn't You Just Call Me John?' The title comes from the difficulty that we 'normal people' face. What should we call people who are autistic or have learning difficulties – the old 'feeble-minded'? A senior lady in the learning disability world asked a group of men for whom she was responsible: how would they like to be called – clients? patients? tenants? or was a person with a learning disability OK? "What should I call you?" she asked. There was a pause until one man put up his hand and said "Couldn't you just call me John?" As I talked with the people who help look after people like John nowadays, I became impressed with the current situation. By ending this first book on a positive note, I thought I was summing up what I had learnt whilst writing the second. However, life is never simple. As I finished this first book, I was waiting in the rain in a queue for fish and chips. I got talking with a man of around sixty. He said that he lived in Hildenborough. So I told him about the book. He knew about Princess Christian – his brother-in-law had been there when he was young. So I asked him for his thoughts.

"That 'Care in the Community'. It's OK for some. But it's definitely not OK for others. In the old days, my brother-in-law used to be happy; he felt

Coda: What Happened to the Buildings; and to the 'Boys' and 'Girls'?

secure; he knew where he was in life; and, above all, he liked the structure of his life. He did his bit of gardening in houses round about. He liked that. It made him feel useful. He got up. He washed. He had his breakfast. And so on. It was all organized and he had his friends with him – all the time. Nowadays, he lives in his own flat in Maidstone. He's not really with it. Not that long ago, he turned up at our house. He was in a terrible state – soaking wet and with no proper clothes. He'd got to us by bus and walking somehow. He was desperate. He couldn't understand what was happening to him. He thought he was going to be thrown out of his flat – he was going to have to live on the streets. Eventually, we found out what was happening. He gets government money each week to pay his £20 rent. The trouble was that it all came by GIRO because he hadn't got a bank account. He didn't understand things like that. So by the time he'd got the GIRO cashed, all the £20 had gone and he'd got into debt. The powers that be – I suppose they didn't understand – they were sounding threatening. No one had been helping him. So we sorted it all out. We got him a bank account and it all seems to work now. But, as I say, 'Care in the Community' does not work for everyone. And my brother, who is a policeman, agrees. He says he's always having to deal with cases like this. And policemen are not trained to help people like this – it's not their job. But they try to help. So the 'Care in the Community' thing might be working for some people who are a bit, you know, but as I said, it doesn't work for everyone."

However, perhaps I have to ask you to read the second book and let you make up your own mind.

Footnotes

Difficulties in the Hairdressers

Lorraine Bose, who has run Genesis Hair Salon in the village of Leigh for twenty-five years, has memories of the Princess Christian patients. One day, when her salon had just opened, a young man, clearly with Down's syndrome, walked into the salon and started talking to the customers, all of whom were kind, most realizing he had probably walked from Princess Christian. Lorraine rang the Hospital and they came to collect him. However, some weeks later, he returned and became particularly lively. Lorraine said that it was quite difficult to keep a straight face and continue doing her lady's hair in a responsible way with an exuberant man standing on his head immediately behind her.

A 'Short Sighted' Story

In the 1980s, an optician in Tonbridge, received a call from a very worried senior nurse at Princess Christian. One of her men was creating terrible difficulties and could the optician help. In due course, the nurse and a youngish man with Down's arrived. The optician guessed that, as is often the case with people with Down's, he would be short sighted; and it turned out to be the case. His best distance to view things was about nine inches. The problem was that he loved television. He sat with his head almost touching the screen. This completely infuriated all the other men in the house who could not see what was happening.

There was a happy outcome. The optician provided the man with a pair of glasses and the nurse rang to say everything was now at peace.

How the Book was Written and Acknowledgements

History books are usually compiled using a good deal of primary written or printed material. This book seldom has that advantage. It started with the aim of bringing together some existing, informal notes about the Princess Christian Farm Colony – the Princess Christian Hospital as it became. As well as some useful information which people in Hildenborough gave me, there were the memories of people who had worked at Princess Christian since the 1960s which brought the Hospital and the Farm to life. The project grew and at least some historical documents were found; and even more people talked with me. I have aimed to include all their names in the text and I am most grateful to them all.

So what has emerged is, I hope, more than a look at the Princess Christian experiment – for that is what it was for a good part of its life – but an illustration of how attitudes to people we nowaday say have learning difficulties have matured from pre-Victorian times until 1995. These changes included advances in medical treatment; but they also include a change of attitude towards people whom the Victorians had called in that gentle phrase 'the Feeble- Minded'.

While I have been lucky to find a range of sources, I feel sad that it has not been easy to talk to the many of the main people that the book is about – the 'colonists' and their successors at the Princess Christian Hospital. How did they feel about their lives in an institution – however humane it was? I did attempt to talk with some who had been at Princess Christian twenty-five or thirty years ago. Most did not really remember but a few said – rather vaguely – 'it was nice'.

I have come to the conclusion that the people of Hildenborough and the surrounding area can be proud to have had such a landmark within the community; and the outside world can think highly of the care given to the 'colonists' (the 'inmates' or the 'patients' or whatever they were called in a particular era) by both the dedicated staff and by the community itself. And, on the whole, the West Kent area can feel that nowadays those with learning disabilities are, almost all as far as I have seen, being looked after with great care – in spite of all the inherent difficulties. As President Kennedy said, "One of the highest achievements of a civilization is the way in which it cares for its handicapped members". The way that our society – each one of us – treats those who are 'a bit different from us' is immensely important.

I have used information from Hildenborough website and Wikipedia; but my particular thanks to Robin Ballard whose father, Bob, was the Engineer at the Hospital from 1947/48 until around 1981; and to Sue Gorman of the Hildenborough History Society, who had done much initial work on the history of Princess Christian and also unearthed a four page document by Mrs M K E Hume and Mr R Cooper which not only confirmed some of the early developments but more importantly outlined progress in the 1970s. Memories of her childhood from Joy Dolling were wonderful and the descriptions from Nancy Vernet and Janet Court, who played a leading role in the change to 'Care in the Community' have also been invaluable. I had a good number of informative and entertaining conversations with Nan Connor and her daughter Nina; and a range of doctors, including John Ford, Adam Skinner and his indomitable mother, Barbara, together with Ken and Anne Evans were always charming and helpful. I have greatly enjoyed hearing from Bob Duffin, Bill Richardson and Ron Wood, Lorraine Bose, Nancy Ashwell, Monica Cecil, Marion and Ralph Cooke and John Beach. Pat Davies and other members of the Hildenborough History Society are doing a great job in general and gave valuable introductions. I am also grateful to George Harvey for his information about 'Spadework'.

I am very lucky to have had Amanda Hawkes to design the book and to insert endless changes. However, above all, I am grateful to Joyce Field who has worked on this book for over three years, not just doing seemingly endless re-types as more information arrived, but for her finding much information from obscure websites that I could never have found. The book would not have been possible without her.

Appendices

Appendix 1: A Glossary of Historical Terms for 'Madness' [89]

The UK Mental Deficiency Act of 1913 categorized learning disabled people as follows:

Idiots – Persons in whose case there exists mental defectiveness of such a degree that they are unable to guard themselves against common dangers such as traffic or fire.

Imbecile – Persons in whose case there exists mental defectiveness which, though not amounting to idiocy, is yet so pronounced that they are incapable of managing themselves and their affairs or, in the case of children, of being taught to do so.

Feeble-minded – Persons in whose case there exists mental defectiveness which, though not amounting to imbecility, is yet so pronounced that they require care, supervision and control for their own protection or the protection of others. Or, in the case of children, that they appear to be permanently incapable by reason of such defectiveness of receiving proper benefit from instruction in ordinary school.

Moral Defective – Persons in whose case there exists mental defectiveness, coupled with strong vicious and criminal propensities and who require care, supervision and control for the protection of others. These people included unmarried mothers.

Other terms in common use in the past

Cretin was the oldest term, from the French, referring to those with both physical and intellectual incapacity.

Moron referred to an adult with the intellectual development similar to an 8 to 12 year old child.

Retarded came from the Latin retardare, meaning to make slow, delay, keep back. Mental retardation was a general term which covered all levels of learning disability.

Mongolism was a medical term first used by Dr John Langdon Down in the 1860s to identify someone with what became known after the Second World War as Down's syndrome.

Appendix 2: The National Association for Promoting The Welfare of the Feebleminded

As the main text outlines, the Association seems to have been formed in 1895 or 1896. Exact details of when and who formed the Association have not been found. Although the Charity Commission's records have been moved to the National Archives at Kew, the large collection has not been indexed and finding the full details is perhaps not important for this book. There are no books or articles specifically about The Association but it is clear that the subject was in the air. There was apparently a separate charity called 'The National Association for the Care of the Feebleminded', but it seems that at some stage they merged and the two titles seemed interchangeable in later years. There were Government Select Committees and Reports in 1898 and 1904. Another major Government report was published in 1908 – 'the Royal Commission on the Care and Control of the Feebleminded'. (This can be seen on-line – all 580 pages of it). This report led to the Radnor Report which in turn led into the 1913 Mental Deficiency Act which again can be found on the web.

It seems that two of the leading lobbyists and experts in the field, Mary Denby and Ellen Pincent, who were both concerned with the 1908 Royal Commission's Report, were also involved with the National Association, probably from its inception; and Mary Denby (1859-1933) had established her own successful farm colony and hospital for the 'mentally subnormal' in Great Warford, Cheshire in 1902. One article mentions briefly that The Duchess Sutherland was President of the Association.

However, by 1914, the various bodies concerned with the care of the feeble-minded, including The National Association which had been set up to oversee The Princess Christian Farm Colony, were amalgamated into a single body 'The Central Association for Mental Welfare'.

In 1946 there was a further amalgamation with the Central Association becoming part of the new National Association for Mental Health (see book 'Education and The Handicapped 1760-1960').

However, while there are no obvious books or articles about the Association, there are a number of books which relate to it, including:

The Borderland of Imbecility: Medicine, Society and the Fabrication of the Feeble Mind in late Victorian and Edwardian England: by Mark Jackson

Education and the Handicapped 1760-1960 by D G Pritchard

Eugenics, Human Genetics and Human Failings: The Eugenics Society, Its Sources and its Critics in Britain by Pauline M H Mazumdar

Prostitution Prevention and Reform in England 1860-1914 by Dr Paula Bartley

Other mentions occur in the British Medical Journal; and Mary Warnock's 1978 Report on 'Special Educational Needs – The Education of Handicapped Children and Young People' has a useful historical section.

Appendix 3: Census Returns for 1911

The following four pages are reproductions of the only Census available from the Princess Christian Farm Colony.

CENSUS OF ENGLAND AND WALES, 1911.

Name and Surname	Relationship to Head of Family	Age Male	Age Female	Particulars as to Marriage	Children Born Alive	Children Living	Children Died	Profession or Occupation	Industry	Employer/Worker	At Home	Birthplace	Nationality
Hall William Barnes	Head	39		Married 14yrs				Householder trader				Portsmouth Hants	62
Hall Sarah Ellen	Wife		38	Married 15yrs	1	1						Gosport Hants	140
Sturdy Andrew Kath. and Hands		30		Single				488 Malton Workmen of Felt Hands				Stone Hunts	630
Cooke Harry		17		"				Assistant Hand 483 Horse & Farm				Wordsworth Oxon	320
Bleesdale William		18		"				"				Fulham London Sur	070
Sharp Russell Cyril	"	20		"				"				Kenswick North	201
Servant Wilfred Harry	"	21		"				"				Mildred Lincolnshire	250
Barnett Victor Percy	"	24		"				"				Southampton Hants	163
Green Ernest Edward Gibbs	"	21		"				"				Fulham London NW	070
Willis Reid Selwyn	"	17		"				"				Atlanta Jordan	
Hunt Albert	"	17		"				"				Nottingham	51
Mullers Fred A	"	20		"				"				Isla Wight	070
Shelton Herbert	"	20		"				"				Fontana S.S.	036
Nothinson Victor	"	18		"				"				Enfield Midds	070
Pollard John	"	27		"				"				Tunbridge Wells Kent	245
North Stewart	"	22		"				"				Wickham	
Wilmes Wallace	"	20		"				"				Paddington London	070
Lopez William	"	20		"				"				N. Kensington London	
Hunt Chris Richard	"	28		"				"				Orrington Kent	
Giles Inla Spring	"	16		"				"				Clanston Essex	111

Males 19 Females 1 Total 20

NAME AND SURNAME	RELATIONSHIP to Head of Family or position in Institution	AGE last Birthday Males / Females	PARTICULARS as to MARRIAGE	PROFESSION or OCCUPATION of Persons aged ten years and upwards.	BIRTHPLACE of every Person.	NATIONALITY of every Person born in a Foreign Country
Echols John C	Amptd est Inmate	19	Single		Crouch Hill London N	
Pettyjo Chas	"	19	"		Epping Essex	
Brockwell Sidney	"	18	"		St John London SE	
Brick George E	"	16	"		Stoneathene S O	
Adams Albert	"	19	"		Epping Forest	
Abbey Arthur W	"	19	"		Mile End London	
Cumberledge William	"	24	"		Victoria Docks Kent	
Hayes Henry	"	17	"		Unknown	
Crane Alfred	"	20	"		Willesden London	
Riley William	"	17	"		Rendalsham Suffolk	
Britto Mac Jones	"	17	"		Sheffield Yorks	
Ayles William	"	17	"		Sunstead Garden Suburb	
Gibson Walter	"	17	"		Hoxton London	
Giles Philip	"	24	"		Cambridge	
Hale Geo Henry Thos	"	27	"		Bromley	
Milverson Cyril	"	17	"		Burdett Road London	
Matthews Robert	"	17	"		Hilldown London NW	
Reynolds Wm Henry	"	17	"		Kingston Hamburg	
Edgwick Ernest	"	17	"		Lullham Kent	
Esher Arthur	"	12	"		Poplar Kent	
Smith Herbt Ed	"	19	"		Paddington London	
Shepherd Walter	"	20	"			
Howell John Henry	"	15	"		Folkstone Kent	
Ward Edgar Andrew	"	22	"		Barnes Estate London	
Nead George Alfred	"	16	"		Croydon Surrey	
Wilkerson Geo E	"	21	"		Unknown	
Gopt Purnell	"	17	"		Redwood Surry	
Leonard Chas	"	14	"		Sheffield Yorks	
Everett John Henry	"	21	"		Stoakwell Rams SW	
Norman George	"	18	"		South Sheffield Para	

[Continues on page 2.]

NAME AND SURNAME	RELATIONSHIP to Head of Family	AGE Male	AGE Female	PARTICULARS as to MARRIAGE				PROFESSION or OCCUPATION			BIRTHPLACE	NATIONALITY
Taylor Norman	inmate	22		Single							Penrtland Lock	000
Cozo Alfred	"	19		"				441 N.A.F.M 183			Northampton	331
Pedegraus William Geo.	Visitor	32		Married 10 yrs	3	3		Gasten chaman 483 worker			Waterloo Road London	000
Pedegraus Alice	Visitor		38	Married 10 yrs				"			Shirley Litton Essex	V.O

Males: 3 Females: 1 Persons: 4

RELATIONSHIP to Head of Family, or Position in Institution.	NAME AND SURNAME.	AGE last Birthday. Males. Females.	PARTICULARS as to MARRIAGE.	PROFESSION or OCCUPATION of Persons aged ten years and upwards.	BIRTHPLACE of every Person.	NATIONALITY of every Person born in a Foreign Country.

	Males	Females	Persons
Total of page 4	3	1	4
Total of page 3	30		30
Total of page 2	19	1	20
Total of page 1	52	2	54
Total of pages 1 to 4			67

State here the number of rooms in the Institution; count the Kitchen as a room, but do not count scullery, landing, lobby, closet, bathroom, nor warehouse, office, shop:—
If the Institution comprises more than one inhabited building, state for each building.

Kind of Dwelling or Institution (Private House, Tenement, &c.) and Condition as to Common, &c.

Main House
not marked

Number of Rooms: 6 / 8 ✗

	Males	Females	Persons
	27	1	28
	25	1	26

I declare that this Schedule is correctly filled up to the best of my knowledge and belief

Signature: Jeannie Smith
for Sister ...
Mulleo Division
Postal Address Hillsborough ...

Appendix 4: The Future of Leybourne Grange and Princess Christian's by W Cowell, Director of Nursing Services for The Tunbridge Wells Area Health Authority from Autumn 1984 Issue of Spotlight

"I was very pleased to receive a recent invitation from Spotlight's new editorial team to say a few words about the future of the mental handicap unit. I am aware of staff anxiety about the long term future and I hope that this brief summary at least goes some way to clarifying the position as far as the UMG can determine at present. [Mr Cowell does not say what the UMG stood for but it was the NHS's and Kent County Council's Social Services' co-ordinating body for these changes, as presumably his readers knew.] I hope also that staff will take this opportunity to discuss some of the issues with each other and as far as is practical, with individual residents and their relatives. I would like to stress that existing plans are based on the current situation and may be subject to change or delay, depending on individual circumstances. What I have to say therefore is the position as it stands now and reflects what the UMG believe to be the likely course of events over the coming decade.

For some considerable time the national policy for mental handicap services has emphasised the need to replace institutional care with local community services. The command document "Better Services for the Mentally Handicapped" (1979) stressed the desirability of small home-like community based residential facilities and this concept was fully endorsed in the extensively researched 'Jay Report' (1979). Health Authorities have been charged with the task of running down large mental handicap hospitals and setting up in their place appropriate residential and other services within the local boundaries. Our own authority, Tunbridge Wells, is faced with the dual task of gradually scaling down two sizeable hospitals (Leybourne Grange and Princess Christian's) and simultaneously creating a National Health Service residential service for certain of our more dependent residents in the community.

District Health Authorities served by Leybourne and Princess Christian's have set up a Kent District Steering Group to assist in achieving the above objectives. The function of this group is to provide a basis for co-ordinating action in bringing about what is clearly going to be a major task. At the same time the UMG have produced a management control plan for both Leybourne Grange and Princess Christian's. This is essentially a blueprint describing the process by which services at both units can be gradually and realistically reduced as the number of residents declines.

The UMG will be discussing the implications of the management control plan with heads of departments and staff representatives over the coming months. We will urge appropriate managers to keep their staff fully aware and involved. The UMG plans to put out regular bulletins in order that all concerned can be fully up to date with progress and developments.

How will this affect the Residents?
Residents will gradually be moved into new homes in the community as near to existing relatives/friends as possible. Some will go into private care and others to Social Services residential units. Some will remain with the NHS and various plans for these residents are being formulated by the responsible districts. In each case great care will be taken to ensure that each resident's personal and individual needs and desires are fulfilled. Close co-operation with relatives and friends is, of course, essential.

It is estimated that about 70 residents each year will require to be re-housed in order to close both Leybourne Grange and Princess Christian's by December 1995. At present we are on target to achieve the 1984/5 figures. We recognise that the more able are likely to leave first and that we will eventually be caring almost exclusively for more dependent residents. The preparation and training of such residents will obviously be extensive and suitable places may become scarcer. We therefore accept that a decade may be over optimistic and that the timescale for closure could be somewhat longer.

What are the implications for Staff?
As resident numbers decline, the unit's budget will be automatically reduced. Some £10,000 is extracted for each resident who is discharged (or dies). This means that revenue has to be systematically reduced annually. The only feasible way of achieving a revenue reduction is to close villas. Staffing costs must be cut as well as everyday running costs such as water, heating and electricity. Depending on the rate that residents leave, the UMG estimate that two or three villas will be closed each year.

Particular buildings have been earmarked for closure based on their structural condition and taking into account issues such as ground floor accommodation. Various departments are scheduled for early closure whilst others will be gradually scaled down. The UMG are looking very carefully into this aspect in order that minimal disruption occurs for both residents and staff. For instance, we are now scrutinising each staff vacancy which occurs individually before making a decision to replace that member of staff.

Whilst the UMG will make every effort to bring about a planned and gradual run down of services, some disruption and change to the lives of both residents and staff is inevitable.

The UMG will be making the strongest possible case to our District Authority for additional support during what is clearly going to be a challenging and even traumatic era in the history of Leybourne Grange and Princess Christian's. Our new Chairman, Sir John Grugeon and his authority colleagues have already indicated their understanding of this and our District Management Team are, of course, very aware and sympathetic to the complex and sensitive nature of running down a major service.

The future however is not all gloom. Whilst long stay facilities are being gradually phased out, existing community based mental handicap services are in the process of being created. This will offer various employment opportunities for staff of all disciplines and many of our former colleagues have already in fact obtained posts with agencies who are in the very early stages of setting up new services. As far as direct care staff is concerned it is absolutely certain that many more staff will be required to service the new model of care. The background and experience of Nursing Staff will of course be of immense value in setting up these new ventures.

Staff Training
What is not so clear is the future pattern of training for direct care staff. One assumes that some change in the present Nurse Training structure is inevitable with the closing of large hospitals. At present active discussions are in progress about the possibility of some form of joint training arrangement between the two statutory bodies and this seems to me to be a logical line to pursue. Whatever is eventually agreed however, qualified and/or experienced Nursing Staff can feel confident that their knowledge and skills will be in great demand in creating a new future for mentally handicapped people.

Summary
During the last hundred years mental handicap hospitals have provided the backbone of residential services for mentally handicapped people. Anyone with any knowledge of these hospitals would not seriously contest the general principle that they are inappropriate places for mentally handicapped people to live and learn. They have nevertheless performed a magnificent job over a considerable time span in the most difficult, frustrating and trying conditions one could possibly conceive. The staff of these hospitals can be justly proud of the task they have performed and of

the exceptional progress which has been achieved in spite of the conditions and against a backlog of public apathy and consistent Government neglect.

It is now recognised and generally accepted that mentally handicapped people have as much right to live in a normal home in the general community as anyone else. Mental handicap is essentially a problem of slow learning rather than ill-health and in this respect large and isolated hospitals are hardly the best place for people to become conversant with normal patterns of living.

Community care however is still in its infancy and is to a large extent untried and untested. It is right that we should now be concentrating our thoughts and efforts on creating a better future for our residents and we will do this with as much skill and sensitivity as possible. Staff of all disciplines and at all levels can assist in the successful outcome, of what will be a massive undertaking, by being positive and realistic about the reasons for, and the motivation of, this undertaking. I am confident that the staff at Leybourne Grange and Princess Christian's will be equal to the task."

Appendix 5: Princess Christian Staff Names Post 1945

This list is given in part to pay tribute to all the staff whose names are known for their work at Princess Christian. However, it includes only a small proportion of those who worked there and it would be good to have more names and dates for future editions.

Superintendents and later Senior Nursing Officers

Miss Jeannie Lewin Fry	?1907/8-?1915
Miss Pitman	?1915-1949
Thalia Koskina, Sister-in-Charge	ca. 1930
S Russell	1949-?1953
Sydney Rymall	?1953-1957
Mr Edward 'Ted' Mason, Chief Male Nurse and later Superintendent	1957-1959
Joe Kenyon	1959-1972
Jack Lobb, Deputy to Superintendent	?1970s
Jim Bell, Senior Nursing Officer	1973-1990
Roy Cooper, Nursing Officer	c1973-1980s
Fred Gardener, Nursing Officer	1970s
Robert Corp (Chief Executive of the Mental Handicap NHS Trust (Leybourne and Princess Christian)	1980-1992
Rob Stevens, Nursing Officer	end 1980s – closure

The Princess Christian Farm Colony and Hospital 1895–1995

Farm Managers
Bill Hobden probably after 1945 – early 1960s
Mr R Palmer early 1960s – late 1970s
John 'Jack' Clayton late 1970s – late 1980s

Tractor Drivers/Farm Workers
Fred Gardener 'Garnie', Tractor Driver 1950s-1960s
Don Perrin, Tractor Driver 1960s-1980s
Charlie Coomber, poultry man 1960s
John Coomber, poultry man/
   tractor driver 1960s
John 'Jack' Clayton, poultry man/
   tractor driver late 1960s – late 1970s
Felix and Mrs Robinson,
   who looked after poultry
Gordon and Sam, Milking Parlour
Don Perrin, Alan Bowen, Fred Gardener,
   farm helpers 1960s – late 1990s

Gardeners
William Moore 1920s and early 1930s
Alf Pooley (lived at North Cottage,
   Riding Lane) 1950s – early 1960s
Jack Leach (lived at Club Cottages,
   Riding Lane) 1960s
Roger Batchelor c 1960s
Bert Woodhams c 1960s
Bob Caffyn (lived at South Cottage,
   Riding Lane) 1970s
Adam Skinner 1975 (temporary)
Danny Gould 1970s

Hospital Engineer
Bob Ballard plus help from
   bricklayer, carpenter, painter, etc 1948-1980
Alan Fellows (Assisted Bob Ballard
   with major projects)

Maintenance
Ernie Kennard, bricklayer 1950s – 1970s
Ron Bennett, painter 1950s – 1960s (for various short periods)
Stan Pargeter, painter 1960s – 1980s

Frank Wooley, carpenter   1960s
Alan Hawkins, carpenter   1968-1972
Ken Fever, carpenter   1970s
Fred Ayling, stoke/maintenance man   1970s/1980s
Keith George, engineering assistant
Terry Cooper, painter
Danny Gould, painter

Cleaning
Vic Martineti (supervisor)
Jimmy Rapa
John Sheaghan
Margaret Mardell

Administrator
Don Cat and Mr Porter   1950s
Charles Porter   1950s – 1960s
Geraldine Stokes   1960s
Simon Bently   c1967
Don Catt (stores)   1960s – late 1970s
Marion Cooke   1973-1990
Elizabeth Myers
Simoon Smith   1980s
But 'Malcolm' is called Administrator in   1984

Catering/Domestic Staff
Mr Kraft (lived Chestnuts) Chef   early 1950s
Dave Bonn   ? 1970s
Ted Harris   1960s – 1980s
Bob Brown   1960s
Danny Gould (trainee who went
  on to nursing)
Ron Buckley   1960s – 1970s
Kathleen Chaplin (originally a resident
  but who graduated to helping
  oversee the kitchen in Glen House)   1960s
Annie Crosby
Jill and John 'Jack' Taylor
Mrs Harris
Jane Davies

The Princess Christian Farm Colony and Hospital 1895–1995

Drivers

Mr Jordan	1960s
Freddie Gould	1970s ?
Monty Coleman	1980s
? Sam	retired after many years, 1982
? Bill	

Nursing Staff: Ward Sisters/Nursing Managers/Charge Nurses etc

Oast House	Pat Tyghe, charge nurse	1960s
Oast House	Ken Fisher, charge nurse	1960s
Oast House	Mr Tickner, charge nurse	1960s
Oast House	Ruth Galligan, ward sister	c1980s
Farm Villa	Cecil Hibbert, charge nurse	1950s
Farm Villa	Mr Redman, charge nurse	1960s
Farm Villa	John Watson, charge nurse	1970s
Farm Villa	Mrs Pat Tynan, charge nurse	1980s
Farm Villa	Harry Hughes, charge nurse	1980s
Alexander House and the Oast	Pat (Paddy) Griffin, charge nurse	1970s – 1990
Alexander House	Harold Neasham, charge nurse	1950s – early 1960
Alexander House	Dai Payne, charge nurse	1960s-1970s
Alexander House	Mr Vigor, charge nurse	1960s
Alexander House	Harry Spencer, charge nurse	1970s
Alexander House	Nina Brannan, ward manager	1987 – 1990/91
Glen House	Nan Connor, ward sister	1958-1991
Glen House	Ms Humphrey, ward sister	early 1950s
Glen House	Mrs Kraft, deputy sister	early 1950s
Glen House	Mrs Russell, staff nurse	1960s
Glen House	Nurse Dobell, ward sister	?1970-1980s
Glen House	Ursula Taylor, ward sister	late 1980s
Glen House	Nurse Black, night staff	1960s
Glen House	Isabel Docking, staff nurse	1970s
Glen House	Mary Beech, staff sister	1977 – 1988

Other Nursing Staff and Assistants

Miss Mitchell, Glen House, residential care assistant	1950/1960
Mrs Blaney, Glen House, residential care assistant	1950/1960
I J Price, sister	1950s
A T Price, nursing assistant	1950s

Appendices

Mrs Kennard, ? nursing assistant	1950s
Mrs Powell, ? nursing assistant	1950s
Miss R Cross, ? nursing assistant	1950s
Mr Pargitter ?nurse	1960s
H.R.H. Hughes is mentioned in 1984, seemingly in charge of staff	
Charles Billington, around early 1980s – title unclear but perhaps a Senior Charge Nurse	
Pam Thompson	
Ken Fisher, charge nurse	around 1979
Harry Spencer, charge nurse	?1980s
John Watson, charge nurse	?1980s
Tom Bowden, charge nurse (?nights)	?1980s
Mrs Dockin, staff nurse	?1980s
Kath Feaver, nurse	c1980
Liz Sherlock, staff nurse	1980s
Mrs Craft, deputy sister	?1980s
Margaret Nye	early 1980-early 2000s
Kelly Holmes, Care Assistant	1987
Deirdre Morgan and sister, Care Assistant	1980s
Marion Crook, care assistant	
Gloria Lyons and daughter, Sharon, care assistant	c1980s
Joyce Hunter, nursing assistant	
Dawn Watson, nursing assistant	
Nobby Clarke	
Mrs Humphrey, nursing assistant	
Mr Hunter, nursing assistant	
Marion Kinchen, nursing assistant, nights	
Mr Docking, nursing assistant, nights	
Isabel Adams, nursing assistant, nights	
Tom, Pam and Isabel who seem to have been nursing staff (who cooked at a barbecue in 1984)	
Alan Hughes, charge nurse, nights	
Tom Bowden, charge nurse, nights	
Cathy Sullivan, night staff	1980s
Greg Brittain, night staff	1980s
Betty Bower, night staff	1980s
Mr & Mrs John Page	late 1970s
Rosa Brooker	1980s
Alison Shorten	late 1980s
Pam Owen	Late 1980s

The Princess Christian Farm Colony and Hospital 1895–1995

Occupational Therapy
Mr Trevors	1960s
Dorothy Vines	1960s
Mrs Humphries	1960s
Marilyn Pettit	for much of 1970s and 1980s
Isabel Adams	1980s
Charlie Buss	
Mrs Carolyn Schweitzer	1987
Ann Trigg (area head of OT, Leybourne)	1980s
Marion Cooke, nurse	
Joan Jenner, nurse	

House Wardens
Nancy Vernet (Assistant Warden at The Farm Cottage)	1986-end 1990s
David .... (Warden at The Farm Cottage)	1980s and 1990s

Teaching 'the girls' (needlework, laundry, etc)
Wynne Woodgate	c1960s/1970s
Joyce Ballard, sewing room	1970s – 1980s
Mrs Buckley, sewing room	1970s

Hairdressing
Mrs Bill Hobden
Selma Cooke

Entertainment
Billy Carcary (mainly 1990s)

Outside GPs/Specialists
Dr Basil Davison	late 1930s until early 1960s
Dr Peter Skinner	early 1960s until mid-1970
Dr Bill Callum (with Dr Ken Evans/ Dr Brian Glaisher and Dr John Kelynack)	mid-1970 until 1990s
Cecile Gorney (psychologist)	late 1980s

Psychiatrist from Leybourne
Dr Peter Anger	c1970s – 1980s

Appendices

Appendix 6: Princess Christian Material in the Kent Archive

The information below about the material on Princess Christian kept in the Kent Archive is given partly in case other researchers wish to refer to them but more to indicate the almost complete lack of information that I have found. There are 115 items about Leybourne Grange but few have direct relevance to Princess Christian (see below). In many cases the material seems to have reached the Archive by mistake and seems entirely random. Clearly they were not officially deposited by the NHS or Kent County Council. However, the main Princess Christian documents are five issues of SPOTLIGHT, the in-house Leybourne Grange and Princess Christian magazine.

Spotlight Autumn 1978 }
Spotlight Autumn 1980 }
Spotlight Summer 1984 }   MH/TW1/AS3/2
Spotlight Winter 1984/5 }
Spotlight Autumn 1984   U4004/6

There is one other paper where Princess Christian is mentioned: FO/Z2/C13/9

Leybourne Grange Material
Minutes of Kent County Council Mental Deficiency Committee 1914-1930: CC/MC/27/1/1
Minutes of Kent County Council Mental Deficiency Committee 1930-1948: CC/MC/271/2 through to 27/1/20
Leybourne Grange Sub Committee: CC/MC/27/2/1
B Series Maps 1932 deposited with the Ministry of Health 1932: C/A8p/227
Instrument of Government for Hospital Special Schools 1982: C/E/28/15/10
"Contact". Internal news sheet of Leybourne Grange 1975-1985: MH/TW1/AS3/1
Leybourne Grange Hospital, West Malling 1967-1984
    General group reference number: U4004
Management audit of nursing Dec 1976 (but maybe only one unit for Leybourne): U/4004/5
Management Meeting Minutes 6 issues 1975-1983: MH/TW1/A53/2

Notes

Chapter 1: What's in a Name?

[1] Professor Pinker is the Canadian born cognitive scientist, psychologist and linguist, currently at Harvard, who has written extensively, including the book "How the Mind Works".

[2] There are two associations which provide advice for families who need to know about Down's syndrome (the National Down Society (NDSS) and the Down's Syndrome Association). They disagree about whether it is Down's syndrome or Down syndrome. I have used the first, not least because that is the spelling used by the NHS. (It is apparently acceptable to say someone has Down's or is a Down's man/woman).

[3] See the Langdon Down Museum and Mencap websites

[4] For example see quotes from The Maidstone Community Mental Handicap Team in 'The Grapevine', the magazine for Leybourne Grange and Princess Christian Vol. 37 No. 2. April 1987

[5] I have added West's Disorder as an early example of a specialized medical term because, firstly, it has lasted a hundred and fifty years and, secondly, it has a local connection. Dr West was a respected Tonbridge doctor whose son, E J West, was plainly mentally ill. He was sent to the Earlswood Mental Asylum under the care of Dr John Langdon-Down in 1860 and his condition given a name. He died of TB with Dr Langdon-Down and the matron at his bedside. [Information from Dr John Ford, Tonbridge medical historian. For further details see Journal of Medical Biography Vol II May 2003 pp. 107-113]. I have not included a large number of medical words which denote difficulties which concern more physical problems. Just look at some of those beginning with 'A'. There are Agnosia, Alexia, Amnesia, Aphasia, Aphemia, Aphonia, Anosmia, Appraxia, Ataxia and so on!

Notes

Chapter 2: From the Start of an Idea to the Second World War

[6] 'Victoria's Daughters', by Jerrold M Packard: publ. Sutton 1998 ISBN 075092568X

[7] All this correspondence and a large amount of other documentation are in the London Metropolitan Archive

[8] 'Victoria's Daughters', by Jerrold M Packard: publ. Sutton 1998 ISBN 075092568X

[9] 'Victoria's Daughters', by Jerrold M Packard: publ. Sutton 1998 ISBN 075092568X, p. 195

[10] Madeleine Rooff gives the founding date as 1895 in her book 'Voluntary Societies and Social Policy' (1957 International Library of Sociology Book Series) although most other sources say 1896.

[11] The Times 10 July 1910

[12] British Medical Journal 14 July 1900 reporting on the AGM 9 July and Madeleine Rooff book mentioned above.

[13] Courier Article 7 May 1920

[14] Murphy 1991, quoted by Nina Brannan (see later in the text) in her University thesis.

[15] Quoted from "Human Traces" by Sebastian Faulks, published Hutchinson 2005 ISBN 978009945826. See in particular pages 70-125.

[16] The Barming Asylum, according to one contemporary description, was said to be in thirty-seven acres looking over the Medway valley with fields covered in hop plantations and woods on park-like hills.

[17] Quoted in "Human Traces" by Sebastian Faulkes, published Hutchinson 2005 ISBN 978009945826.

[18] The double-barrelled surname of 'Langdon-Down' was adopted by John Langdon Haydon Down later in his life. In some documents it is shown as hyphenated, in some not. For the sake of consistency the hyphenated surname is used in this book when referring to family members.

[19] From "Neurotribes" by Steve Silberman pages 164/5. Allen and Unwin ISBN 978-1-76011-3636. 534 pages.

[20] Source: Hildenborough History Society's notes which say that Lord Derby of Knowsley provided the land. The Society also has details of the extent of the land owned by Lord Derby in the area.

21. An informal document, with much useful information, kindly provided by the Hildenborough History Society

22. Cambridge University Alumni 1261-1900 via Ancestry.com

23. See obituary in Morning Post 26 April 1878.

24. In the 1891 Census she is at the London Hospital

25. See 1901 Census for Normansfield Licensed House for the Reception of Imbeciles, Teddington.

26. The Charity Commission do not keep their historical records which in some cases have been passed to the National Archive at Kew. However, the registration of the National Association has not been found at Kew.

27. Although a national census was taken every ten years from 1841, census data is only available to the public after a hundred years. There are, therefore, no census details available for Normansfield or Princess Christian after 1911.

28. See www.langdondownmuseum.org.uk

29. Mary Langdon-Down's letters are held in the London Metropolitan Archives.

30. Comparisons of the value of money from earlier times are often very misleading. The website www.measuringworth.com uses three criteria to measure the relative value of income or wealth over time. So the *Historic Standard of Living* system, £20,000 in 1896 is reckoned to be in the region of £2,067,000 in 2014; the *Economic Status* system values the sum to be in the region of £14,050,000; and the *Economic Power* value is said to be in the region of £23,000,000. Whichever system is used, Dr John died rich – almost certainly mainly due to his Harley Street practice.

31. The figures for Normansfield come largely from a study done by U3A students on the 1868-1913 papers given on the Langdon Down museum website. The full figures for the length of stay at Normansfield are 31% for more than ten years, 13% six to ten years, 13% three to five years, 20% one to two years, and 19% less than a year. See www.langdondownmuseum.org.uk. It is worth noting that there was very little inflation over this period, so figures for wages etc would have stayed much the same in the 1868 to 1913 period.

32. It is particularly galling that, according to the curator of the Langdon Down Museum at Normansfield, Ian Healy-Jones, the extensive archive of Normansfield has no mention of the Princess Christian Farm Colony. (Indeed, Healy-Jones had never heard of it.) This is strange when forty years of work at Normansfield was clearly the basis for the successful Princess Christian Farm Colony.

Notes

[33] See the book "Clough Williams-Ellis" by Richard Haslam, publ. RIBA. Drawings Monograph No. 2 p. 29.

[34] The confirmation that the house was bought from Lord Derby comes from the present owners, Liz and Mark Smith.

[35] Several newspaper articles from around 1932 including one from the Tonbridge Free Press seems to indicate that Oaklands was being used as some sort of international centre. Source: Robin Ballard, son of the engineer at the Farm Colony post World War Two.

[36] Source: Hildenborough History Society

[37] Sevenoaks Chronicle & Kentish Advertiser 11 March 1910

[38] Hildenborough History Society papers

[39] A copy of a map was kindly supplied by Mrs Janet Richardson, a cartographer and past Chairman of the Hildenborough History Society. It is dated March 1867 and is part of the Ordnance Plan of the Parish of Tunbridge Hundred and Washlingstone, in the County of Kent (Western Division). It was published by Colonel Sir Henry Jones RE and surveyed by Captain Palmer RE. Scale 1:2500. It is available in the Leigh Historical Society archive.

[40] Sevenoaks Chronicle & Kentish Advertiser 29 April 1910

[41] From the 1921/22 Annual Report and Accounts of the National Association

[42] 3 May 1912

[43] 7 June 1912 Sevenoaks Chronicle & Kentish Advertiser

[44] From the 1871 Census, a column was included to show whether people were 'deaf and dumb', 'blind', 'imbecile/idiot' or 'lunatics'. By the time of the 1901 census the term 'feeble-minded' was also included grouped with 'imbecile'. The age at which the person was afflicted was also included. A quick scan of the 1871 census for the village of Leigh shows a few 'deaf and dumb' and 'blind' but no one in the imbecile or lunatic category. In the 1901 census, Leigh did have one feeble-minded person. But in any case, many households might not mention that a member of the family was 'slow', etc.

[45] Sevenoaks Chronicle & Kentish Advertiser 11 March 1910

[46] Sevenoaks Chronicle & Kentish Advertiser 11 March 1910

[47] Sevenoaks Chronicle & Kentish Advertiser 29 April 1910

48. By 1920, there were 2,783 unmarried females in mental hospitals or workhouses because they were deemed to be "mentally defective" – and pregnant. See 'Sinners? Scroungers? Saints? Unmarried Motherhood in the Twentieth Century' by Pat Thane and Tanya Evans. Published 2013 by OUP. ISBN 13 978-0199681983

49. Information as well as plans from RIBA Library

50. Sevenoaks Chronicle 2 July 1926

51. The Minutes of the 1921/22 Annual Report and Accounts give fuller details; and the Colony had a sub-committee which oversaw who should be admitted.

52. The Minutes of the 1921/22 Annual Report and Accounts also mention how concerned the Association was about the lack of places there were in the country for severely mentally ill people that the Association was not set up to help.

53. Archive numbers CC/MC/27/1/1 and CC/MC/27/2/1. The first has nothing of relevance; the second has the various instances some of which are given in the main text.

54. The Minutes of the 1921/22 Annual Report and Accounts have been found by the Hildenborough History Society and copies of them are held in their archive.

55. Kent & Sussex Courier 20 January 1922

56. From 1921/22 Annual Report and Accounts which gives full lists of the numerous Committees. The papers can be seen in the Hildenborough History Society archives.

57. Sevenoaks Chronicle & Kentish Advertiser 2 July 1926

58. From Hildenborough Men's Club Minutes Books 1924 to 1935

59. Sevenoaks Chronicle & Kentish Advertiser 30 September 1938

Chapter 3: From the Second World War until the early 1980s

60. The Nursing Mirror Magazine 1952

61. Documents provided by the charity *mcch*, with particular thanks to Karen Read, their recently retired Director of Operations who started her career at Leybourne. Other details come largely from a Kent Messenger Special Report of June 1973 and from the Kent Archive (see Appendix 10)

62. See also the 1972/73 White Paper "Better Services for the Mentally Handicapped"

63. The Kent Messenger Special Report of June 1973, mentioned in note 61.

64. Taken from Nina Connor's University thesis.

Notes

[65] Again the quotes are taken from the Kent Messenger Special Supplement on Leybourne, published June 1973 which was given to the author by *mcch* and which can be seen in full at the Kent Archive.

[66] Information from Mrs Elaine Knight who later befriended Derek when he was moved to Tonbridge.

[67] Mr Mason was the Hospital's Superintendent. Joy Dolling's younger brother, Roger, had become close friends with Mr Mason's son, Geoff. It was through the late Geoff Mason that the article from the Nursing Mirror was obtained.

[68] The Nursing Mirror article includes these photographs.

[69] The Vicars at St. John's during the era of the Princess Christian Farm Colony/Hospital:
Rev James Stone 1901-1918
Rev H J Warde 1918-1924
Rev L G Chamberlen MC MA 1924-1934
Rev E H Wade MA 1934-1935
Rev W H Bass MA BD 1935-1939
Rev E N E Fraser AKC 1939-1951
Rev A R Fountain 1951-1959
Rev P. Tadman 1960-1962
Rev P S Plunket MA TCD 1962-1968
Rev G A R Swannell 1968-1980
Rev D R Corfe 1982-1990
Rev Robert Bawtree 1991-2004

[70] Source: 1983 Report by the Development Team for Tunbridge Wells Health Authority – unpublished but kindly unearthed by Maidstone and Tunbridge Wells NHS Trust Library

[71] From Spotlight, Winter 1984/85, the Leybourne Grange Magazine. Kent Archive MH/TWI/AS 3/2.

[72] Kent Archive ref. MH/TW1/AS3/2. However, it should be noted that very few documents in the Kent Archives or the Tonbridge Archives have any relevance to the Princess Christian Hospital.

[73] Nicholas Willsher of the King's Fund has looked up the Hospital Year Books for the post war period. The relative lack of importance of the Princess Christian Hospital is perhaps indicated by the lack of information given in the Year Books. Entries are only given until 1978 and, even then, only the number of beds and the name of the Senior Officer for 1972-1974, J. Kenyon, SRN RNMS (SNO). Nan Connor's memory of the number of beds is confirmed with 200 beds in 1972/73 gradually decreasing to 176 in 1978, the last year of any information.

74. Sending unmarried mothers who were deemed defective to a mental institution was allowed under the 1913 Mental Deficiency Act. Instances were still occasionally happening fifty years later. See 'Sinners? Scroungers? Saints? Unmarried Motherhood in the Twentieth Century' by Pat and Tanya Evans. Publ. OUP 2013, 240 pages, ISBN 13978-0199681983

Chapter 4: Moving Towards the Closure of Princess Christian

75. The full Report is held in the Leigh & District Historical Society archive.

76. Two Wessex scales were developed by the Wessex Regional Hospital Board, Winchester. See Albert Kushlick, Roger Blunden and Gillian Cox papers from the Maidstone & Tunbridge Wells Hospital Board. (https:// contents.bjdd.net/oldPDFs/5588to96.pdf)

77. From the Kent & Sussex Courier 2 October 1987

78. The actual dates when the Princess Christian Trust bought buildings and land vary in different sources. The details in this section come from an undated and unattributed note, probably written around 1992/3 and supplied by the Hildenborough History Society.

79. News in Focus: September 29 and 30 1987 'Down on the Farm'

80. From The Newspaper of the Kent Social Services Number 13, Feb 1988

81. 'Black, White and Gold', first published in 2005 by Virgin Books but updated and in paperback 2008. ISBN 9780753513170.

82. From the unpublished Report for the Tunbridge Wells Health Authority kindly and informally provided by the Maidstone & Tunbridge Wells Health Authority Library.

83. The author has not been able to find out what WTEs are – although he has asked various NHS experts.

84. As per note 83.

85. The Grapevine, Journal of Leybourne Grange and Princess Christian's April 1987 Vol. 37 No. 3, supplied by MCCH

86. This last point meant the local NHS authorities no longer had to pay for the upkeep of that particular man or woman from Princess Christian. Additionally, they could – as they did – sell the various sites for substantial sums. As an indication of how far the £11,700 would have gone to help the Social Services departments not only find staffing costs but also to buy, build or rent new sheltered accommodation in Tonbridge or Hildenborough in the

Notes

1985 – 1991 period, a two-bedroom flat would have cost £45,000 (mortgages were over 11%) or a rental cost of around £1,800 a year. A four-bedroom house cost around £140,000 with an annual rent being around £5,600. (Figures from Tim O'Neill, partner of Langford Rae O'Neill). So the £45,000 for four Princess Christian residents would have gone a reasonable way to help finance staffing and housing costs – in Year One at least.

Chapter 5: Coda: What Happened To The Buildings; and to the 'Boys' and 'Girls'?

[87] Seven detached houses, fifteen terraced houses, four semi-detached houses, one maisonette and one apartment block and one bungalow, plus two houses in the rebuilt Oast House. Details from Phil White, Chairman of the Residents' Association.

[88] From 'Neurotribes' by Steve Silberman, p. 338.

Appendix 1

[89] See www.langdondownmuseum.org.uk

Gorman, Sue 172
Gorney, Cecile 150
Gosling, F R (police) 54
Grant, David 132-134, 137
Great Forge Farm 165
Griffin, Bill 137-140, 149
Groombridges (undertakers) 102
Grugeon, Sir John 121-122
Guys Hospital 86

Hadlow College 161
Harrow School 19
Harley Street – consulting room 19, 24, 51
Harvey, George 172
Hawkes, Amanda (iv), 172
Heath, Ted 68
Helena Victoria (Princess Christian's daughter) 52
Hilden Brook 42, 92
Hilden Brook Farm 157
Hildenborough, C of E Primary School 73
Hildenborough Church – see St John's Church
Hildenborough Cricket Club 72, 83-84
Hildenborough GP Practice 118
Hildenborough Men's Club 59
Hildenborough Vestry minutes 33
Hildenborough Youth Club 84
Hillman Minx (car) 75
Hobden, Bill 61, 77, 91
Hollenden, Lord 75
Holmes, Dame Kelly (vii) 126-127
Horsfield, G 109
Hostel, The 104
Hubble, Mr (farm) 165
Hulett, J 109
Hume, Mrs M K E 93, 109, 111, 172

Ingram, Richard and Julie 158

Jackson, Daisy 45

KCC Social Services 5, 52, 72, 76, 121, 132, 142, 154
Kelynack, Dr John 85
Kennedy, John (President, USA) (vii), 172

Kent Archive 46, 94
Kent & Sussex Hospital 86
Kent County Council (KCC) 5, 121-123, 152, 154, 161
Kent County Council Mental Deficiency Committee 46-47
Kent County Show 147
Kent Messenger 71
Kenyon, Joe 83, 99, 100
Knotley Hall 144-145

LAMPS (Local Amateur Dramatic Society) 107
Land Army, girls 59, 61
Langdon-Down family 15-18, 21, 25, 159
    Dr John Langdon-Down 3, 16, 22, 24, 144, 166
    Mary (née Crellin, wife of above) 16, 20-22, 109
    Dr Reginald (son of above) 16-17, 20-22, 24, 26, 32, 49, 51, 58, 109, 144
    Jane (wife, née Cleveland) 18-19, 51
    Ruth (wife, née Turnbull) 18-19, 51, 53, 57, 157
    Dr Percival (son of Dr John) 16-17, 20, 24, 26
    Helen (wife of Dr Percival) 26-27
    Stella 26, 32, 51, 52
    Elspie 26, 32, 51
    John ('Jack') 32, 51
    Norman 27
    Anthony ('Tony') 59, 109, 111, 144, 165, 167
    Joseph 15
    Hannah 15
League of Friends 150, 107-112, 144, 165
Leybourne Grange Hospital 46, 55, 62, 66-71, 76, 84-85, 88, 92, 94, 102, 106, 117, 129, 131-132, 138, 149, 164
London Hospital 15, 19-20, 24
Lones, Francis 44
Lunacy Commission 13

Maidstone Community Health Trust 144
Maidstone Community Mental Handicap Team 131, 137
Maidstone & Tunbridge Wells NHS Trust 117, 138
Manley, Rev C A 49

Index

Marie-Louise Princess (daughter of Princess Christian) 47-48, 52
Margaret, Princess 101
Mason, Edward 76-77, 81, 83, 90
McNeil, Bill 121-122
Meals on Wheels 162
Mental Capacity Act 2005 159
Mental Deficiency Act 1959 71-72
Merrow Down, Surrey (houses) 31
Milk round 33, 42, 47, 101
Mill Lane 92, 109
Mongolism, Mongol 16, 32, 51, 89
Moore, R 78
Moore, William Stephen 54
Morgan, Deirdre 126
Myers, Elizabeth 105

National Association for Promoting The Welfare of The Feeble Minded (see 'National Association')
National Association 12, 17-18, 20, 32, 35-38, 44-45, 48, 52, 56, 58-59, 159, 174-175
National Association's 1921/22 Annual Report 43, 45, 48-51, 62
National Trust 31
Neasham, Harold 73, 81
Nelson, Lord 147
Neve, Arthur (Coroner) 53-54
New College, Oxford 52
New Trench Farm 18, 32, 18, 44
Newson, Tommy 123
Nicholls, Irene 124
Nightingale, Florence 12
Normansfield 16, 19-22, 24, 27, 32, 45, 51, 59, 76
North and South Cottages 141
Nursing Mirror 75-82

Oaklands (later Alexander house) 26-27, 58-59, 61
Oakwood Hospital, Barming (see Barming Asylum/Hospital)
Oast House 26, 28-29, 44, 72, 80-82, 102, 104, 126
Oast House Villa 113
Occupational Therapy 93, 125, 141
"Of Human Traces" – novel 14
Old Barn 109

Orpington 35
Oxford Street 75

Packard (car) 75
Palmer, R 91
Pargitter, Mr 148
Parry Morgan, Miss G 109
Perrin, Don 91
Perry, Mary 93
Pembury Hospital, Tunbridge Wells 102, 153
Pepenbury 168
Pinker, Prof. Stephen 2
Pitman Hall 49, 56, 87, 100-101, 107-110
Pitman, Miss 33, 43, 46, 47, 49-52, 56, 60-61
Plas Brondanw 31
Plaxtol Saw Mill 101
Plough, The (Pub in Powder Mill Lane) 99-100
Portmeirion 26, 30, 31
Prader-Willi syndrome 4
Pratt, Stephen 124
Princess Christian – see Christian, Princess
Princess Christian Hospital, Weymouth 12
Princess Helena 52
Princess Marie-Louise 47-48, 52

Rattenbury, Thomas 53-54
Regents Street 75
Retts syndrome 4
Richardson, Bill 33, 93, 134, 144-166, 172
Richardson, Janet 93
Rochester, Bishop of 37, 47, 56
Rooke, Charles Alexander 34
Royal Free Hospital 11
Rutherford, Margaret 61
Russell, S 81, 83
Ryall, Mr 83

Sackville-West of Knole 18
Sadler, Tony 101
St John's Church, Hildenborough 50, 87, 90, 162
St Mary's Road, Tonbridge 82
St Thomas Hospital 11
Scott, James 26
Scott, Jill 109, 136
Scott Project 109

Seagrave, William and Alice 34
Sevenoaks Council 49
Sevenoaks Fatstock and Sale Show 124
Sevenoaks Guardians of the Poor 49
Sewing Room 80
Sherlock, Liz 99
Sherwood House 141
Singer Gazelle 75, 86
Skinner, Dr Adam 85-86, 88, 136, 168, 172
Skinner, Barbara 85, 172
Skinner, Dr Peter 85, 88, 102-103, 136, 147
Skinner, Quentin 87
Smith, F 54
Social Club 87, 107-109
Southern, Penny 164
Spadework 138, 154-155, 172
'Spastic' 163
Spender, Eric 166
Steward-Green (architects) 54
Stone Lodge 73-74

Taylor, Brian and Gillian 87, 162
Taylor, Ursula 84, 108
Thomas, Danny 124
Tidby, Rosemary 155, 163
Tonbridge Amateur Dramatic Society 50
Tonbridge Fatstock Show 50
Tonbridge Gunpowder Mills Site 95
Tonbridge Market 72
Tonbridge School 108
Trench House 80
Trigg, Ann 119-120
Trinity College, Cambridge 19-20, 31
Tull, Edward and Sarah 34
Tunbridge Wells 35
Tunbridge Wells Health Authority 121, 153
Turkey Mill, Maidstone 55
Turnbull, Ruth (see Mrs Reginald Langdon-Down)
Turnbull, Evelyn 19, 51, 53

U3A Study 22, 24
Upper Hollanden Farm 18, 37, 82

VAD Hospital 51, 53
Vernet, Nancy 144-148, 172

Victoria, Queen 1, 11
Victorians, The 3, 89
Vidler, Mrs 109
Vietnam War 69
Vines Lane 73-74, 91-92
VSU (Voluntary Service Unit) 71, 105, 108, 135, 149, 165

Warde, Rev H J 50
Warders, GP Practice 95
Wardill, H R 58
Weald of Kent NHS Community Health Trust 140, 143
Welbeck St, Consulting Room 19, 51
Wessex Scale 118-119
West's Disorder 6
Westwell Asylum 46
Wiggins, Rev Karl 87
Willard, Dick 46
Williams, Esther 100
Williams syndrome 4
Williams-Ellis, Bertram Clough 26, 30-31, 34, 37-43, 81
Wilmore, Bert 109-110
WRVS 162
Wood, Ron 33, 134, 164-166, 172
Woodgate, Wynne 165